Manual of Oocyte Retrieval and Preparation in Human Assisted Reproduction

Manual of Oocyte Retrieval and Preparation in Human Assisted Reproduction

Edited by

Rachel Cutting
Human Fertilisation and Embryology Authority, London

Mostafa Metwally
Royal Hallamshire Hospital, Sheffield

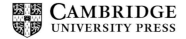

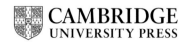

Shaftesbury Road, Cambridge CB2 8BS, United Kingdom

One Liberty Plaza, 20th Floor, New York, NY 10006, USA

477 Williamstown Road, Port Melbourne, VIC 3207, Australia

314–321, 3rd Floor, Plot 3, Splendor Forum, Jasola District Centre,
New Delhi – 110025, India

103 Penang Road, #05–06/07, Visioncrest Commercial, Singapore
238467

Cambridge University Press is part of Cambridge University Press
& Assessment, a department of the University of Cambridge.

We share the University's mission to contribute to society through
the pursuit of education, learning and research at the highest
international levels of excellence.

www.cambridge.org
Information on this title: www.cambridge.org/9781108799690

DOI: 10.1017/9781108891646

© Cambridge University Press & Assessment 2023

First published 2023

*A catalogue record for this publication is available from the British
Library.*

ISBN 978-1-108-79969-0 Paperback

....

Every effort has been made in preparing this book to provide
accurate and up-to-date information that is in accord with accepted
standards and practice at the time of publication. Although case
histories are drawn from actual cases, every effort has been made to
disguise the identities of the individuals involved. Nevertheless, the
authors, editors, and publishers can make no warranties that the
information contained herein is totally free from error, not least
because clinical standards are constantly changing through research
and regulation. The authors, editors, and publishers therefore dis-
claim all liability for direct or consequential damages resulting from
the use of material contained in this book. Readers are strongly
advised to pay careful attention to information provided by the
manufacturer of any drugs or equipment that they plan to use.

Contents

Color plates are to be found between pages 57 and 58.

Contributors

Valentine Akande, Bristol Centre for Reproductive Medicine, 135 Aztec W, Almondsbury, Bristol BS32 4UB, UK. Email: Valentine@FertilityBristol.com

Basak Balaban, Assisted Reproduction Unit, VKF American Hospital Istanbul, Turkey. Email: basak-b@amerikanhastanesi.org

Kate Brian, Fertility Network UK, Trafalgar Rd, London SE10 9EQ, UK. Email: kate@fertilitynetworkuk.org

Rachel Cutting, Jessop Fertility, Tree Root Walk, Sheffield Teaching Hospital NHS Foundation Trust, Sheffield S10 2SF, UK. Email: rachel.cutting@sth.nhs.uk

Stephen Davies (retired), The Jessop Wing and Royal Hallamshire Hospital, The University of Sheffield, Tree Root Walk, Sheffield S10 3HY, UK.

Andrew Drakeley, Liverpool Women's NHS Foundation Trust, Crown Street, Liverpool L8 7SS, UK; Edge Hill University, St Helens Rd, Ormskirk L39 4QP, UK. Email: adrakeley@yahoo.com

Thomas Ebner, Kepler University, Kinderwunsch Zentrum, Linz, Austria. Email: Thomas.Ebner@kepleruniklinikum.at

Mark A. Fenwick, Academic Unit of Reproductive and Developmental Medicine, Department of Oncology and Metabolism, University of Sheffield, Beech Hill Road, Sheffield S10 2RX, UK. Email: m.a.fenwick@sheffield.ac.uk

Stephen Harbottle, Cambridge IVF, Maris Lane, Trumpington, Cambridge CB2 9LG, UK. Email: stephen.harbottle@addenbrookes.nhs.uk

Hajeb Kamali, Bristol Centre for Reproductive Medicine, 135 Aztec W, Almondsbury, Bristol BS32 4UB, UK. Email: hajeb.kamali@doctors.org.uk

İpek Keles, Assisted Reproduction Unit, VKF Koc University Hospital Istanbul, Turkey. Email: ikeles@-kuh.ku.edu.tr

Peter I. Kerecsenyi, Manchester Fertility, Amelia House, Cheadle Royal Business Park, 3 Oakwood Square, Cheshire, Cheadle SK8 3SB, UK. Email: peter@manchesterfertility.com

Sarah J. Martins da Silva, Reproductive and Developmental Biology, Ninewells Hospital and Medical School, University of Dundee, Dundee DD1 9SY, UK. Email: s.martinsdasilva@dundee.ac.uk

Raj Mathur, Manchester University NHS Foundation Trust, Oxford Road, Manchester M13 9WL, UK. Email: rmathur@nhs.net

Alison McTavish, Aberdeen Fertility Centre, University of Aberdeen, Aberdeen, UK. Email: a.r.mctavish@abdn.ac.uk

Mostafa Metwally, The Jessop Wing and Royal Hallamshire Hospital, University of Sheffield, Tree Root Walk, Sheffield S10 3HY, UK. Email: mmetwally@nhs.net

Lewis Nancarrow, Hewitt Fertility Centre, Liverpool Women's NHS Foundation Trust, Crown Street, Liverpool L8 7SS, UK. Email: lewis.nancarrow@doctors.org.uk

Lukasz Polanski, Guy's Hospital, Great Maze Pond, London SE1 9RT, UK. Email: Lucas.polanski@hotmail.com

Alka Prakash, Cambridge IVF, Kefford House, Maris Lane, Trumpington, Cambridge CB2 9LG, UK. Email: alkaprakash@hotmail.com

Jennifer M. Ulyatt, Assisted Conception Unit, Ninewells Hospital, Dundee DD1 9SY, UK. Email: jennifer.ulyatt@nhs.scot

Lucy Wood, Jessop Fertility, Tree Root Walk, Sheffield Teaching Hospital NHS Foundation Trust, Sheffield S10 2SF, UK. Email: lucy.wood@sth.nhs.uk

Bryan Woodward, X&Y Fertility, 144a New Walk, Leicester LE1 7JA, UK. Email: theeggman68@gmail.com

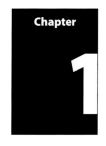

Chapter

1

The Ovary: A General Overview of Follicle Formation and Development

Mark A. Fenwick

1.1 Introduction

In the context of reproduction, the key functions of the ovary are to provide an environment that supports the maturation of oocytes for ovulation alongside adequate production of sex steroids to prepare for and sustain a potential pregnancy. These functions are not mutually exclusive, as each depends on follicle and oocyte growth and maturation progressing in a coordinated and timely manner. Our current understanding of how the ovary is formed, with its limited supply of follicles, and how individual follicles develop and achieve these functions of oocyte support and steroidogenesis are summarised briefly this chapter.

1.2 Sex Determination and Early Gonadal Development

In humans, male and female embryos are morphologically similar until around week 6 of development when activation of the molecular programme from sex chromosomes allocated at fertilisation sets in motion the formation of a sex-specific gonadal phenotype. Prior to this, a small cluster of pluripotent primordial germ cells (PGCs), first identified in the posterior yolk sac endoderm, begins to proliferate and migrate along the hindgut, through the dorsal mesentery, to eventually settle on either side of the developing aorta in the emerging gonads, or 'gonadal ridges'. This migration of PGCs, driven by chemotactic signals (e.g. KIT/KITLG), occurs alongside proliferation and inward migration of somatic cells to create a bulge on the ventromedial aspect of each mesonephros called the gonadal ridge. The gonadal ridges, covered by coelomic epithelium, develop alongside the two adjacent embryonic ducts, the Wolffian (also known as the mesonephric) and Müllerian (also known as the paramesonephric) ducts, which all together constitute a bipotential reproductive system.

Subsequent differentiation of the gonads is generally dependent on the genetic constitution of the embryo. In males, brief and timely expression of the sex-determining region on the Y chromosome (*SRY* gene) in somatic cells, together with other transcription factors (e.g. SF1 and WT1), drives expression of SRY-box transcription factor 9 (SOX9). This transcription factor in turn activates the expression of an array of genes that drives a pre-Sertoli cell phenotype, including cues that amplify and propagate the molecular programme along adjacent somatic and germ cells (e.g. FGF9 and PTGDS), leading to the differentiation of the fetal testis. PGCs, now called spermatogonia, undergo further proliferation before arresting in mitosis. The production of testosterone from newly differentiated Leydig cell precursors stimulates the Wolffian ducts to develop into components of the male reproductive tract – the vas deferens, epididymis and seminal vesicles – while the production of anti-Müllerian hormone (AMH), driven by SOX9 in pre-Sertoli cells, causes regression of the Müllerian ducts.

Female XX embryos lack *SRY*, and therefore SOX9 expression remains low in somatic cells within the developing gonad. These cells, thought to be derived from the mesenchyme or coelomic epithelium overlying the gonadal ridge, additionally express factors that actively repress SOX9 and its targets. Such factors, including RSPO1, WNT4, CTNNB, FST and FOXL2, are necessary to promote and maintain the differentiation of these cells into 'pre-granulosa' cells. Adequate expression of these proteins is fundamentally important for maintaining the phenotype of this lineage, even into adulthood, with experimental examples of mutations shown to precipitate a partial gonadal sex reversal or the development of an ovotestis phenotype. Secreted signals from the pre-granulosa cells are important for (1) stimulating PGCs (now called oogonia) to arrest in meiosis (see Section 1.3), and (2) promoting differentiation of nearby somatic cells, from an alternative lineage, into 'pre-theca' cells. Thus, the pre-granulosa cells initiate a series of developmental events to define the tissue that will eventually become the ovary. In comparison with the fetal testis, the relatively low levels of testosterone and AMH cause the Wolffian ducts to regress and the Müllerian ducts to persist, the latter of which will form the precursor structures to the oviduct, uterus and upper vagina in the female [1].

1.3 Follicle Formation: Establishment of the Ovarian Reserve

As the fetal ovary is being established, the germ cells – now called oogonia – continue to proliferate by mitosis to form dense oogonial cell clusters; however, cell division is incomplete, and many of the oogonia remain connected to each other with a shared cytoplasm. Retinoic acid, which is produced by the somatic cells of the ovary and the adjacent mesonephros, binds to stimulated by retinoic acid 8 (STRA8) receptors on oogonia to initiate the process of meiosis, while at the same time inhibiting further proliferation of these cells. Oogonia proceed relatively slowly through the early stages of meiosis to arrest in the diplotene stage of prophase I, at which point they are called oocytes. In humans, arrested oocytes are identifiable in fetal ovaries between 10 and 24 weeks of gestation. It is during this time that primordial follicle formation occurs, a process whereby pre-granulosa cells invade and interpose between the germ cells in their clusters to envelop individual oocytes. Germ cells that fail to enter meiosis or become completely encapsulated in pre-granulosa cells degenerate by apoptosis [2].

It is generally believed that the net effect of these mitotic and apoptotic processes throughout this period leads to the final establishment of the ovarian reserve. Based on a relatively small number of histological studies, the average number of follicles in the human ovarian reserve (i.e. in both ovaries) is estimated to be 500,000–1,000,000 at the time of birth [3, 4]. Evidence for *de novo* synthesis of oocytes after this time is still a matter of debate, although recent studies have identified a small population of 'oogonial stem cells' that persist into adulthood, and these can be isolated and differentiated into oocyte-like cells in

vitro [5]. More recent studies in mice have shown that adult somatic cells of non-ovarian lineages can be 'reprogrammed' in vitro to generate new oocytes capable of fertilisation and generation of offspring [6, 7]. Thus, research efforts are being directed towards developing novel fertility preservation strategies through artificial amplification of the ovarian reserve, although the medical potential of these findings is still far from being realised.

1.4 Follicle Development
1.4.1 Primordial Follicles
Primordial follicles, situated in the cortex of the ovary, constitute the most numerous population of follicles at any one time. Each primordial follicle consists of a small, primary oocyte (~20 μm in diameter) arrested in prophase I of meiosis, surrounded by a layer of squamous pre-granulosa cells and enveloped by a basement membrane. Within the oocyte, the nucleus, also known as the germinal vesicle, contains chromosomes in the dictyate state, a configuration conducive for active gene transcription. Both the oocyte and pre-granulosa cells are tightly connected by junctional complexes to allow for bidirectional communication and preservation of a viable, yet relatively quiescent phenotype. Thus, although primordial follicles are often referred to as 'dormant', it is important to note that they are still intrinsically active, with the oocyte and surrounding pre-granulosa cells undergoing normal cellular metabolism and homeostasis.

From the time the reserve is established within the fetal ovary, the number of primordial follicles progressively decreases; in other words, the ovarian reserve begins a steady trajectory of decline. For most females, the main reason why the ovary eventually runs out of follicles is because they are continuously recruited to grow. In adults, this continuous activation eventually leads to the menopause, a natural event that occurs in women at an average age of 51 years, when fewer than 1,000 viable primordial follicles remain. Interestingly, it has been proposed that the initial size of the ovarian reserve formed during fetal development is a predictor of the timing of menopause, as there is a strong association between the rate of follicle loss and the advancement of chronological age [3]. Genetic variation, which can influence the initial size of the ovarian reserve but also the rate of primordial follicle activation, can also impact the timing of menopause, which, if it occurs before the age of 40, is termed premature ovarian insufficiency. Regardless of genetic influence, there is a continuous departure of primordial follicles from the ovarian reserve as they activate and enter a trajectory of irreversible growth. The remaining non-growing primordial follicles may be retained in a relatively quiescent but potentially vulnerable state for up to 40–50 years before being activated. However, this protracted period of suspended animation makes them particularly susceptible to chronic and acute exposures to environmental toxicants. Products of cigarette smoking, diet and alcohol consumption are all lifestyle factors reported to affect the viability or rate of decline of the ovarian reserve. Therefore, it is not only the quantity of primordial follicles that becomes diminished with age but also the quality. This is important in the context of female fertility, especially now that the age of first-time parents has steadily increased over the past 40 years [8].

The question of why some primordial follicles are activated to grow while others stay arrested is a major area of interest in reproductive science and medicine. Numerous molecular signals have been implicated in a range of models; however, an intricate balance of stimulatory and inhibitory factors (e.g. KL, BMP4, BMP7, bFGF, LIF and KGF) along with spatial access to these factors are likely to be important. Transgenic mouse models have established that adequate expression of key transcription factors (e.g. Nobox, Sohlh1, Sohlh2, Foxo3a and Lhx8) are essential for oocyte activation. Studies have also found that AMH, produced by developing preantral follicles, exerts an inhibitory influence on the primordial pool, while factors that activate the PI3K/AKT/mTOR signalling pathways in pre-granulosa cells and oocytes have a stimulatory effect on growth. Identifying how these pathways are regulated in this context is now the subject of many research groups. In most mammalian species, an increase in the rate of pre-/granulosa cell division, accompanied by morphological changes in shape of these cells from a squamous to a cuboidal form, as well as a relatively abrupt increase in oocyte growth, are all morphological features characteristic of follicle activation [9, 10].

1.4.2 Preantral Follicles

Follicles committed to activate and grow eventually establish a tightly packed single layer of cuboidal granulosa cells. Once this layer is complete, these primary-stage follicles require adequate expression of oocyte-derived factors for further development, specifically growth differentiation factor 9 (GDF9) and bone morphogenetic protein 15 (BMP15), members of the transforming growth factor β (TGFβ) family. These molecular signals act on surrounding somatic cells, which in turn signal back to the oocyte – possibly by KIT/KITL – to ensure both cell types develop in synchrony. The oocyte also develops a glycoprotein-rich zona pellucida (ZP) coat, which remains throughout the life of the oocyte. The ZP is important for fertilisation and pre-implantation development and is only shed just prior to implantation. Despite the presence of this relatively thick barrier, granulosa cells develop long thread-like processes, called transzonal projections, which extend through the ZP to the surface of the oocyte where they connect to gap junctions. The existence of gap junctions between the oocyte and granulosa cells, and also between adjacent granulosa cells, is vital for allowing bidirectional molecular communication.

It is also during the primary stage when stromal stem cells begin to differentiate into a layer of theca cells and associate with the basement membrane. As preantral follicle development progresses, granulosa and theca cells continue to proliferate under the influence of local growth factors – principally originating from the oocyte (e.g. GDF9, BMP15) but also from the surrounding cells and tissues. Several signalling pathways play key roles at this stage, including the TGFβ (e.g. activin), insulin-like growth factor (IGF) and epidermal growth factor (EGF) pathways; however, many others are also implicated. The combination of these mitogenic signals causes multilayering of the somatic cells and further growth of the oocyte, leading to overall expansion of the follicle into a secondary-stage or multilayered preantral follicle [11].

Importantly, these early stages of preantral follicle development occur independently of gonadotrophins and steroid hormones. As such, early follicle development occurs throughout pre-pubertal life – even in the fetal ovary – although fetal preantral/small antral follicles will never develop much further due to insufficient levels of follicle-stimulating hormone (FSH). In the post-pubertal ovary, FSH from the pituitary binds to functional FSH receptors expressed on granulosa cells of preantral follicles. FSH augments the actions of local growth factors to mainly stimulate

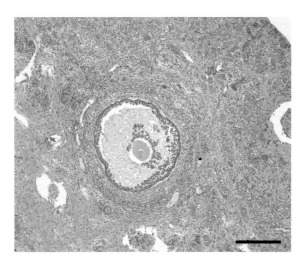

Figure 1.1 The human neonatal ovary. Numerous primordial follicles are embedded in the stroma, and a small antral follicle measuring approximately 400 μm in diameter is evident (centre). Although the antral follicle appears well developed, it is destined to undergo atresia due to insufficient levels of gonadotrophins in early life. Scale bar = 200 μm. A black and white version of this figure will appear in some formats. For the colour version, refer to the plate section. Image kindly provided by Dr Suzannah Williams and Briet Bjarkadottir (University of Oxford).

the rate of follicle growth by promoting cell proliferation and, with further development, stimulates the differentiation of follicle cells to become steroidogenic (see Section 1.4.3.2). Most of the large preantral/small antral follicles that develop when FSH levels are low – for example, before puberty (Figure 1.1), or during the luteal phase of the menstrual cycle – will perish, a process known as atresia. However, in the postpubertal ovary, if the timing is right, around 7–10 follicles per ovary per cycle will be selected for further development to the antral stage.

1.4.3 Antral Follicles

In the human ovary, the developmental journey from a small primordial (0.03 mm/30 μm diameter) to a large preantral follicle (0.2 mm/200 μm) occurs over several months. By comparison, antral follicle development (>200 μm) occurs rapidly over a 6-week time frame, with significant expansion (from 2 to 25 mm) during the final 2 weeks corresponding to the follicular phase of the menstrual cycle. During antral follicle growth, a series of developmental events ensures that the ovary communicates effectively with the hypothalamus and pituitary to set in motion a feedback mechanism with the gonad that regulates the

production of sex steroids to prepare the reproductive tract and coordinate this with ovulation. The following sections provide a brief summary of the developmental changes that occur in the oocyte and somatic compartments as gonadotrophin-dependent follicles develop towards the ovulatory stage.

1.4.3.1 Morphological Changes

As large preantral follicles become increasingly responsive to gonadotrophins, fluid rich in proteins, mostly derived from granulosa cell secretions and serum transudate, begins to appear. These discrete pockets of fluid eventually coalesce into a single, large antrum, which allows unimpeded diffusion of growth factors and molecules. This is important because, while the theca layer is highly vascularised, blood vessels never penetrate the basement membrane of the follicle until ovulation occurs; therefore, granulosa cells and the oocyte are sustained in a nutrient-rich environment despite their relative distance from the vasculature. Granulosa and theca cell proliferation occurs at an increased rate due to the powerful actions of steroid and peptide hormones and local growth factors, although the rapid expansion of the antral follicle throughout the follicular phase of the menstrual cycle occurs mostly as a consequence of the increased antral volume. Within the antral follicle, the granulosa cells differentiate into two specialised types: (1) the cumulus cells surrounding and in direct contact with the fully grown oocyte, and (2) the mural granulosa cells at the periphery of the follicle. Likewise, the theca cells differentiate into two specialised layers: (1) the vascularised theca interna, which is in direct contact with the basement membrane, and (2) the more peripheral theca externa, containing fibroblasts and smooth muscle-like cells, providing structural integrity to the expanding follicle.

1.4.3.2 Steroidogenesis and Atresia

The mural granulosa cells, along with the theca interna cells, are dependent on gonadotrophins for survival and steroidogenesis. The 'two-cell, two-gonadotrophin hypothesis' proposed in the 1970s refers to luteinising hormone (LH) binding and activating the LH receptors (LHRs) expressed on theca interna cells, stimulating production of androgen, while FSH signals via the FSH receptors (FSHRs) on mural granulosa cells to convert androgen to oestrogen [12]. FSHRs and LHRs are G protein-coupled cell-surface receptors that activate second messengers – cyclic adenosine monophosphate (cAMP), which drives protein kinase A (PKA), as well as other kinase pathways – which each signal to the nucleus to drive transcription of target genes. Such targets are varied but include inhibitors of apoptosis, such as the BCL-2 family, which are important for follicle maintenance and survival. Inadequate gonadotrophin signalling in the antral follicle leads to somatic cell death and loss of basement membrane integrity, allowing leukocyte infiltration, collapse of the antrum and eventual oocyte demise. This degenerative process – otherwise known as atresia – is a discrete mechanism resulting in rapid clearance of follicles that are no longer destined for further development. Although atresia can occur at any stage of follicle development, it is predominantly a feature of antral follicles and is more easily recognisable microscopically in larger follicles due the relatively high number of cells. It is estimated that, in humans, atresia accounts for the loss of over 99.9% of the follicles from the original reserve at birth. Therefore, in order for antral follicles to survive, they need to express functional gonadotrophin receptors, particularly for FSH, during the early stages, and LH in the later stages to coincide with the cyclical rise in systemic gonadotrophins.

Of the small proportion of follicles that remain responsive to adequate levels of gonadotrophins (i.e. during the follicular phase of the menstrual cycle), cAMP/PKA signalling also drives the expression of key enzymes involved in growth and steroidogenesis. In theca cells, key steroidogenic enzymes include cholesterol side change cleavage/cytochrome P450 (encoded by the *CYP11A1* gene), which converts cholesterol, derived from the circulation, to pregnenolone within the mitochondria (Figure 1.2). 3-β-Hydroxysteroid dehydrogenase (HSD3B1) then converts pregnenolone to progesterone. Under the action of 17α-hydroxylase/17,20-lyase enzyme (CYP17A1), both pregnenolone and progesterone can be modified to the 17α-hydroxy forms, which are the precursor substrates for the androgens. These are the first rate-limiting steps involved in steroidogenesis.

Progestagens, often referred as the grandparental steroids, are converted to the androgens dehydroepiandrosterone (DHEA) and androstenedione in the presence of CYP17A1. Importantly, 17β-hydroxysteroid dehydrogenase 1 (HSD17B1) converts these androgens into androstenediol and testosterone, respectively. Dihydrotestosterone (DHT), a potent,

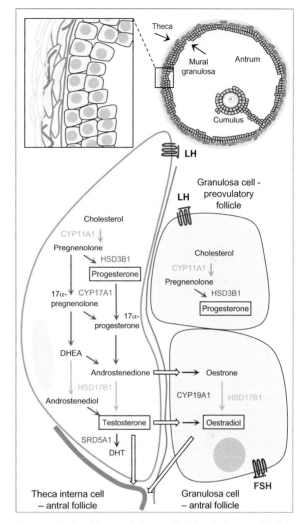

Figure 1.2 Steroid synthesis in antral follicles. During antral follicle development, luteinising hormone (LH) binds to the LH receptor on theca cells, which regulates the expression and activity of key steroidogenic enzymes, allowing the modification of cholesterol into androgens. Testosterone and androstenedione diffuse across the basement membrane where they are converted to oestrogens through the activity of aromatase (CYP19A1), which is regulated by follicle-stimulating hormone (FSH) signalling in granulosa cells. In pre-ovulatory follicles, LH receptor is also expressed in granulosa cells to further amplify progesterone synthesis. Note: steroidogenic enzymes are presented as protein symbols (refer to main text for protein name) with corresponding coloured arrows indicating enzyme activity. A black and white version of this figure will appear in some formats. For the colour version, refer to the plate section.

non-aromatisable androgen, is also produced from the activity of 5α-reductase 1 (SRD5A1) on testosterone. Additionally, both DHEA and androstenediol can be further converted by HSD3B1 to androstenedione and testosterone, respectively, both of which are the precursor substrates for the oestrogens. These substrates, being lipophilic steroids, are able to readily diffuse through the basement membrane into the adjacent granulosa cells.

Although theca cells are capable of producing small amounts of oestrogens, granulosa cells fundamentally lack the enzyme (i.e. CYP17A1) required to produce the androgenic substrates. Instead, FSH/FSHR signalling in granulosa cells drives aromatase (CYP19A1) activity, which enables conversion of the theca-derived, aromatisable steroids androstenedione and testosterone to oestrogens. Here, oestradiol-17β is derived from aromatisation of testosterone, or through conversion of oestrone by HSD17B1. Oestradiol is the major form of oestrogen secreted back across the basement membrane into the theca interna where it enters the circulation through the large blood vessels [13, 14].

Although steroid hormones are fundamentally important for endocrine signalling throughout the body, both steroid and peptide hormones have important roles in further enhancing antral follicle development. Androgens from the theca, along with FSH, as well as oestrogens from the granulosa cells, all stimulate the further proliferation of granulosa cells. Androgens also promote aromatase activity, together creating a positive-feedback mechanism to significantly increase oestrogen output during the follicular phase of the cycle [15]. Other growth factors, such as IGF-1 and other TGFβ members (e.g. activins, inhibins and follistatin), are produced in response to gonadotrophin signalling and are also implicated in increasing the rate of granulosa and theca cell proliferation. FSH also causes elevated expression of inhibin B (inhibin α and βB heterodimer), while both FSH and LH promote the expression of inhibin A (inhibin α and βA heterodimer); thus, as follicle development proceeds, the elevated ratio of inhibin A: inhibin B along with rising oestrogen in the blood can be used as markers of follicle expansion. Inhibins and oestrogens are also important for supressing FSH, a feedback mechanism that causes a shift in hormonal support during the latter half of the follicular phase. In the human menstrual cycle, this results in regression of subsidiary follicles, allowing a single follicle to go on to ovulation (see Section 1.4.4).

1.4.3.3 Oocyte Development

Although the oocyte is arrested in the first prophase of meiosis throughout preantral and antral follicle development, it is far from inactive. Oocyte growth continues throughout the preantral stage to reach a maximum size of around 120 μm in small antral follicles. During this time, the oocyte synthesises and accumulates a vast amount of RNA – approximately $200\times$ more relative to a somatic cell. Much of the mRNA is actively transcribed and polyadenylated for translation in a stage-dependent manner as the oocyte develops and becomes competent to resume meiosis; however, many mRNAs are also transcribed and deadenylated for degradation or storage towards the end of follicle development, a process indispensable for development into a viable embryo. During antral follicle development, the oocyte also begins to synthesise the machinery required for further meiotic progression. Maturation-promoting factor (MPF), a protein complex involving cyclin-dependent kinase (CDK) and cyclin B, is produced to enable meiotic progression but is held in abeyance by high levels of cAMP. The relationship between the oocyte and the adjacent granulosa cells is crucial for the maintenance of cAMP. This is because granulosa cells provide a source of cyclic guanosine monophosphate (cGMP) via gap junctions to inhibit the activity of phosphodiesterase (PDE3A), an enzyme that acts to degrade cAMP (see Section 1.4.4.2) [16].

1.4.4 The Ovulatory Follicle

In mono-ovulatory species such as humans, usually only one antral follicle will continue to develop to the pre-ovulatory stage. Although the mechanism for this selection is not yet fully understood, it is thought that follicles that produce comparatively high levels of IGF and the receptor IGFR1, in response to both FSH activity and oocyte signals, exhibit augmented steroidogenesis, which in turn supports a rapid advancement of follicle growth. The elevated levels of oestrogen produced by the pre-ovulatory follicle eventually promote LHR expression in the mural granulosa cells. Oestrogens entering the circulation also alter the activity of gonadotropin-releasing hormone-expressing neurons in the hypothalamus, resulting in a surge of LH secretion from the pituitary. These acutely high levels of circulating LH bind to LHR in the pre-ovulatory follicle to initiate a host of events in the lead up to ovulation 24–36 hours later. The following sections summarise the key changes that occur in the follicle and oocyte during that time.

1.4.4.1 Cumulus Expansion

Throughout antral follicle development, cumulus cells surrounding the oocyte are fairly closely packed, forming a unit known as the cumulus–oocyte complex (COC). Within a few hours of the LH surge, the cumulus cells surrounding the oocyte loosen and the COC undergoes rapid expansion. This process is precipitated by the elevation in LH signalling in mural granulosa cells, which drives expression of EGF-like factors (amphiregulin, epiregulin), which are secreted into the antrum to bind EGF receptors located on cumulus cells. These EGF-like signals, along with growth factors secreted from the oocyte (e.g. GDF9, BMP15 and others) provide a powerful cocktail of stimulants that promotes the upregulation of genes necessary for rapid proliferation and differentiation (e.g. *HAS2*, *PTGS2*, *PTX3* and *TNFAIP6*) of cumulus cells, which, in turn, secrete a gel-like matrix of hyaluronan and stabilisation factors causing expansion. This expanded cumulus is important for nourishment of the oocyte and the embryo during the peri-conception period, and also aids in oocyte pick-up by the Fallopian tube [15, 17].

1.4.4.2 Resumption of Meiosis

As the cumulus expands, the gap junctions/transzonal projections between the oocyte and surrounding cells close. This loss of cGMP source from the granulosa cells allows PDE3A activation and cAMP degradation in the oocyte. The consequential reduction in cAMP causes dephosphorylation of CDK1 and activation of MPF to enable meiosis to resume. Microscopically, the changes can be visualised by the breakdown of the germinal vesicle envelope (also known as germinal vesicle breakdown), formation and assembly of the meiotic spindle (enabling chromosomal segregation), formation of cortical granules towards the periphery of the oocyte and the subsequent extrusion of the first polar body following completion of the first meiotic division. A cytostatic factor then blocks MPF causing the oocyte to arrest again, this time in metaphase II. New proteins are then synthesised to prepare for the completion of meiosis to produce a haploid gamete for fertilisation [15, 16].

1.4.4.3 Ovulation

In the mural granulosa cells, as well as production of EGF-like factors, LHR signalling drives expression of steroidogenic enzymes (CYP11A1, HSD3B1) to enable the production of progesterone. The mural granulosa cells lose the ability to respond to oestrogens and instead the LH and progesterone stimulate mitogenesis and further progesterone synthesis. Although the elevation in progesterone is essential for ovulation to occur, it is also believed to depress the growth of less mature follicles, thus enabling dominance of a pre-ovulatory follicle. The actions of progesterone lead to considerable expansion of the pre-ovulatory follicle and cause it to bulge from the ovarian surface with a relatively thin layer of granulosa and theca cells. This thin layer, called the stigma, is avascular and is subject to the progesterone-stimulated activities of proteolytic enzymes such as matrix metalloproteinases (MMPs), tissue inhibitors of MMPs, plasminogen activator and cyclo-oxygenase/prostaglandins. The internal pressure of the follicle along with the contractile activity of the theca externa results in follicle rupture, leading to expulsion of follicular fluid and the COC around 24–36 hours after the LH surge [13].

1.5 Corpus Luteum

Following ovulation, the basement membrane of the follicle collapses and is breached by invading blood vessels. The loss of oocyte-derived factors along with the LH-induced promotion of steroidogenesis causes the remaining granulosa and theca cells to differentiate into large and small lutein cells, respectively. Both cells continue to produce progesterone, but androgens, oestrogens, oxytocin and inhibin A are also produced by the corpus luteum. The initial action of LH along with the paracrine activity of progesterone provides luteotrophic support to allow the structure to persist until pregnancy occurs, at which point human chorionic gonadotrophin from the developing conceptus replaces LH. If no pregnancy occurs, the loss of peptide hormone signalling and the progressive reduction in progesterone is associated with luteal regression towards the end of the menstrual cycle, with reabsorption of the corpus luteum [18].

1.6 Summary

The ovary is an incredibly dynamic organ: from the time it is formed in the fetus and right throughout adult reproductive life, there is constant remodelling (Figure 1.3). The activity of specific transcription factors drives the differentiation of somatic and germ cells, which become arranged into the basic germ cell units – the primordial follicles. From this precious reserve, a proportion of follicles are constantly being

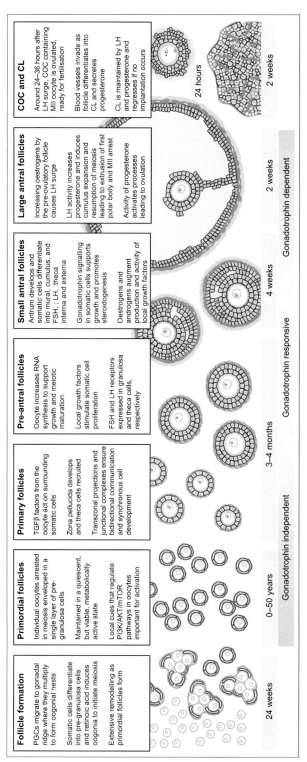

Follicle formation

PGCs migrate to gonadal ridge where they multiply to form oogonial nests

Somatic cells differentiate into pre-granulosa cells and retinoic acid induces oogonia to initiate meiosis

Extensive remodelling as primordial follicles form

24 weeks

Gonadotrophin independent

Primordial follicles

Individual oocytes arrested in meiosis enveloped in a single layer of pre-granulosa cells

Maintained in a quiescent, but viable, metabolically active state

Local cues that regulate PI3K/AKT/mTOR pathways in oocytes important for activation

0–50 years

Gonadotrophin independent

Primary follicles

TGFβ factors from the oocyte act on surrounding somatic cells

Zona pellucida develops and theca cells recruited

Transzonal projections and junctional complexes ensure bidirectional communication and synchronous cell development

3–4 months

Gonadotrophin responsive

Pre-antral follicles

Oocyte increases RNA synthesis to support growth and meiotic maturation

Local growth factors stimulate somatic cell proliferation

FSH and LH receptors expressed in granulosa and theca cells, respectively

2 weeks

Gonadotrophin responsive

Small antral follicles

Antrum develops and somatic cells differentiate into mural, cumulus, and FSH₁; LH₁ theca interna and externa

Gonadotrophin signalling in somatic cells supports growth and promotes steroidogenesis

Oestrogens and androgens augment production and activity of local growth factors

4 weeks

Gonadotrophin dependent

Large antral follicles

Increasing oestrogens by the pre-ovulatory follicle causes LH surge

LH activity increases progesterone and induces cumulus expansion and resumption of meiosis leading to extrusion of first polar body and MII arrest

Activity of progesterone activates processes leading to ovulation

2 weeks

Gonadotrophin dependent

COC and CL

Around 24–36 hours after LH surge, COC containing MII oocyte is ovulated, ready for fertilisation

Blood vessels invade as follicle differentiates into CL and secretes progesterone

CL is maintained by LH and progesterone and regresses if no implantation occurs

24 hours

2 weeks

Figure 1.3 Summary of germ cell development from follicle formation to ovulation. Key stage-specific events are indicated in the text boxes. CL, corpus luteum; FSH, follicle-stimulating hormone; LH, luteinising hormone; MII, metaphase II. A black and white version of this figure will appear in some formats. For the colour version, refer to the plate section.

activated to grow, a process driven by local cues and involving timely activity of cell-specific signals. Further development throughout the preantral stages depends on synchronous growth of the oocyte and somatic cells, which progressively become responsive and eventually dependent on the timely rise in gonadotrophins from the pituitary. Throughout the process, the developmental and maturational changes in the oocyte, granulosa and theca cells are critical determinants in ensuring the production of sex steroids and eventually the release of a mature metaphase II oocyte at the time of ovulation. The surrounding cells and structures, which have not been discussed here but include the vasculature, lymphatics and nerves, all set within stroma and encased by a surface epithelium, must also cope with the ongoing demands of internal restructuring. The complexity of these interactions in time and space is fundamental for ovarian function and female fertility.

Acknowledgements

The author wishes to thank Professor Kate Hardy and Professor Stephen Franks (Imperial College London) for reading and commenting on the text, and Dr Suzannah Williams and Briet Bjarkadottir (University of Oxford) for kindly providing the image used in Figure 1.1.

References

1. She ZY, Yang WX. *Sry* and *SoxE* genes: how they participate in mammalian sex determination and gonadal development? *Semin Cell Dev Biol* 2017;**63**, 13–22. doi: 10.1016/j. semcdb.2016.07.032

2. Wang C, Zhou B, Xia G. Mechanisms controlling germline cyst breakdown and primordial follicle formation. *Cell Mol Life Sci* 2017;**74**(14):2547–66. doi: 10.1007/s00018-017-2480-6

3. Wallace WH, Kelsey TW. Human ovarian reserve from conception to the menopause. *PLoS One* 2010;**5**(1):e8772. doi: 10.1371/ journal.pone.0008772

4. Hansen KR, Knowlton NS, Thyer AC, et al. A new model of reproductive aging: the decline in ovarian non-growing follicle number from birth to menopause. *Hum Reprod* 2008;**23** (3):699–708. doi: 10.1093/ humrep/dem408

5. White YA, Woods DC, Takai Y, et al. Oocyte formation by mitotically active germ cells purified from ovaries of reproductive-age women. *Nat Med* 2012;**18**(3):413–21. doi: 10.1038/nm.2669

6. Tian C, Liu L, Ye X, et al. Functional oocytes derived from granulosa cells. *Cell Rep* 2019;**29** (13):4256–67.e9. doi: 10.1016/j. celrep.2019.11.080

7. Hikabe O, Hamazaki N, Nagamatsu G, et al. Reconstitution in vitro of the entire cycle of the mouse female germ line. *Nature* 2016;**539** (7628):299–303. doi: 10.1038/ nature20104

8. Nelson SM, Telfer EE, Anderson RA. The ageing ovary and uterus: new biological insights. *Hum Reprod Update* 2013;**19**(1):67–83. doi: 10.1093/humupd/dms043

9. Kallen A, Polotsky AJ, Johnson J. Untapped reserves: controlling primordial follicle growth activation. *Trends Mol Med* 2018;**24**(3):319–31. doi: 10.1016/j. molmed.2018.01.008

10. Ford EA, Beckett EL, Roman SD, McLaughlin EA, Sutherland JM. Advances in human primordial follicle activation and premature ovarian insufficiency. *Reproduction* 2020;**159**(1): R15–29. doi: 10.1530/REP-19-0201

11. Edson MA, Nagaraja AK, Matzuk MM. The mammalian ovary from genesis to revelation. *Endocr Rev* 2009;**30**(6):624–712. doi: 10.1210/ er.2009-0012

12. Hillier SG, Whitelaw PF, Smyth CD. Follicular oestrogen synthesis: the 'two-cell, two-gonadotrophin' model revisited. *Mol Cell Endocrinol* 1994;**100** (1–2):51–4. doi: 10.1016/0303-7207(94)90278-x

13. Duffy DM, Ko CM, Jo M, Brannstrom M, Curry TE. Ovulation: parallels with inflammatory processes. *Endocr Rev* 2019;**40**(2):369–416. doi: 10.1210/er.2018-00075

14. Palermo R. Differential actions of FSH and LH during folliculogenesis. *Reprod Biomed Online* 2007;**15**(3):326–37. doi: 10.1016/s1472-6483(10)60347-1

15. Sánchez F, Smitz J. Molecular control of oogenesis. *Biochim Biophys Acta* 2012;**1822** (12):1896–912. doi: 10.1016/j. bbadis.2012.05.013

16. Jaffe LA, Egbert JR. Regulation of mammalian oocyte meiosis by intercellular communication within the ovarian follicle. *Annu Rev Physiol* 2017;**79**:237–60. doi: 10.1146/ annurev-physiol-022516-034102

17. Robker RL, Hennebold JD, Russell DL. Coordination of ovulation and oocyte maturation: a good egg at the right time. *Endocrinology* 2018;**159**(9):3209–18. doi: 10.1210/en.2018-00485

18. Stouffer RL, Bishop CV, Bogan RL, Xu F, Hennebold JD. Endocrine and local control of the primate corpus luteum. *Reprod Biol* 2013;**13**(4):259–71. doi: 10.1016/j.repbio.2013.08.002

Monitoring of Ovarian Stimulation

Lewis Nancarrow and Andrew Drakeley

2.1 Introduction

Monitoring of ovarian stimulation plays a key role in the recruitment of mature oocytes, which in turn leads to better fertilisation rates and embryo development.

The main aim of clinicians is to ensure that sufficiently mature oocytes are collected to achieve a pregnancy, while not overstimulating the ovaries, which can lead to the potentially fatal condition of ovarian hyperstimulation syndrome (OHSS). The emphasis for fertility clinics is controlled ovarian stimulation (COS).

Following the first successful in vitro fertilisation (IVF) cycle in 1978, original monitoring of ovarian stimulation was based on multiple daily urinary or serum oestrogen or pregnandiol levels. This method continued in the early years of IVF, moving more to oestradiol profiles, although when used alone this resulted in up to 40% of collections having only immature oocytes [1]. This was due to oestrogen levels varying for the number of follicles and not necessarily being associated with follicle maturity, leading to premature triggering and follicle aspiration.

Current practice for COS predominantly uses transvaginal ultrasonography with or without hormonal testing. This allows clinicians to adjust stimulation doses depending on the patient's response or even to cancel a cycle where the response has been inadequate or excessive. Regular monitoring of COS determines the appropriate timing for final trigger injection, and identification of those at risk of OHSS and implementation of interventions to reduce the likelihood of developing OHSS. Routine monitoring of COS cycles will normally begin anywhere from day 6 of gonadotrophin stimulation and will then be repeated every 2–3 days thereafter until significant follicular maturity has been achieved.

Oestradiol monitoring during ovarian stimulation can be used as an adjunct to ultrasound to help clarify decision making. Follicles less than 10 mm in mean diameter produce very small amounts of measurable oestradiol, whereas those that are greater than 10 mm will produce progressively more oestradiol as they enlarge and mature. Oestradiol levels will rise exponentially during COS with levels excreted from maturing follicles doubling every 2–3 days. In a natural ovulatory cycle, oestradiol levels peak at between 730 and 1,470 pmol/l, just before the luteinising hormone (LH) surge [2]. These levels can be transferred to COS cycles, and levels of oestradiol can be correlated against the number of follicles present. If levels of oestradiol remain below 730 pmol/l, the likelihood of pregnancy is low, and if levels remain static or are reducing, then this is an indication to consider cancelling the cycle. Levels between 1,835 and 5,506 pmol/l are when best results are achieved; however, levels may peak higher than this if there are more follicles. If levels of oestradiol exceed 11,000 pmol/l, this can act as an alert to the clinician of the risk of the patient developing OHSS. However, if a patient has polycystic ovaries, they may have higher baseline oestradiol levels and this needs to be taken into account when monitoring stimulation based on the patient's hormone profile.

Ultrasound monitoring throughout COS is essential for the management of most patients. Scanning at the beginning of the cycle helps to identify whether there are any pathologies that may hinder ovarian stimulation, such as ovarian cysts, and counting of small antral follicles can also allow adaptation of the initial dose of gonadotrophin to ensure a better response. Repeat monitoring can be commenced after 6 days of stimulation and can help determine the number of follicles recruited. Adjustment in gonadotrophin dosing can be implemented at this point if necessary; for example, if all follicles remain less than

10 mm in diameter, then an increase in the dose could be recommended and is done so in some treatment centres. However, some studies have shown that adjustment of gonadotrophin dose midway through the cycle results in poorer oocyte numbers and pregnancy rates, begging the question of whether it is necessary to make changes during a stimulation cycle and whether is it necessary to scan mid-stimulation if changes are not to be of benefit.

A day 6 scan can offer reassurance to a patient with regard to their progress and also makes them feel that they are getting additional/better care. However, this is another appointment for patients to arrange, at an additional cost to either the treatment centre or the patient themselves. Sometimes a balance needs to be struck between fewer patient visits and a belief of being better looked after.

Scans can otherwise be repeated at day 9 or 10 of stimulation and then every 2–3 days thereafter if the response is poor or excessive, depending on unit practice. Once follicles have reached a certain level of maturity (>17 mm in diameter), this is an indication for the maturation trigger injection. If follicles are less than 15 mm or greater than 24 mm, then the chance of obtaining good-quality oocytes and subsequently achieving a pregnancy is reduced [3]. Between 11 and 12 days of stimulation is more likely to yield more oocytes of optimal maturity; however, patient responses to gonadotrophins will inevitably vary, with some requiring only 9 days of stimulation and other patients requiring a more prolonged course of gonadotrophins. There is a reduction in pregnancy rates when stimulation is less than 8 days or more than 13 days (34% decrease in pregnancy rates at >13 days of stimulation), but those with polycystic ovaries are the exception, with a longer duration of stimulation resulting in pregnancies even after 18 days of stimulation [4].

Follicular measurements are best achieved by the mean of the two largest orthogonal measurements of the follicle. Single diameters of the follicles are more unreliable in a stimulated cycle, as the follicles are often deformed by adjacent follicular growth; therefore, a mean of the two diameters will give a more reliable result. It has been shown that there is only a slight difference between the mean of two diameters in comparison with three (−0.3 mm) and therefore it is more efficient to determine the mean size of the follicle based on the two measurements. However, with ultrasound, the reproducibility of follicle diameters is mediocre, with intraoperative variability of ±2 or ±3 mm highlighting the need for improvement in this area.

Current advances in ultrasound, particularly three-dimensional (3D) measurements of follicular size, may lead to quicker and easier determination of follicular maturity and reduce the likelihood of operator variability, which is inherent with two-dimensional mean diameter measurements. With most newer scan machines having the capability to perform 3D imaging and follicular measurements, this may become a tool used more frequently for ovarian stimulation monitoring and could potentially lead to an improvement in oocyte maturity and quality, although more studies involving 3D follicular monitoring are required to determine this.

The use of hormonal monitoring in COS is debatable and varies among units as to whether to include these additional tests. A meta-analysis reviewing differences between ultrasound monitoring alone versus ultrasound and hormonal monitoring failed to show any significant difference between oocyte numbers collected, clinical pregnancy rates and cases of OHSS [5]. However, this interpretation was limited by the imprecision of the findings and the overall low quality of the included studies [5].

Additional hormonal testing adds costs to both clinicians and patients, with potential delays on management decisions depending on the results of the tests. Performing additional hormonal testing may also require extra appointments, which may add to an already busy clinic workload, while patients may find additional appointments another stress in their treatment process when coordinating their appointment with their own working commitments.

However, recent studies have looked into the monitoring of progesterone levels in the late follicular phase of ovarian stimulation and its effect on assisted reproductive technology success rates. The review by Lawrenz et al. highlighted the issues that can occur with premature progesterone rises and the impact that these have on both endometrial receptivity and embryo development [6]. Gene receptivity and expression were monitored from endometrial biopsies and compared from natural and stimulated cycles. In comparison with the natural cycles, those that had a raised progesterone level showed increased upregulation and downregulation in genes thought to be involved with endometrial receptivity, and a number of studies in the review noticed reduced pregnancy and implantation rates in those whose progesterone level was greater than 1 ng/ml, with more significant differences seen as the progesterone level increased. On reviewing embryo development, there was no difference between fertilisation rate and blastulation rate; however, the total number of top-quality blastocysts was significantly reduced in the group with raised progesterone.

Administration of corticosteroids during stimulation has been shown to prevent premature progesterone rises, as well as other considerations such as not prolonging ovarian stimulation, using a stepdown approach of stimulation with corifollitropin-α as opposed to daily follicle-stimulating hormone (FSH) injections or freezing all embryos created in cycles with a significant early progesterone rise. A minority of patients might see a significant LH fall on first commencing use of gonadotropin-releasing hormone (GnRH) antagonists mid-stimulation, but more work is needed to assess whether routine testing for this phenomenon is useful.

The review by Lawrenz et al. identified the significance of progesterone levels and the effect they have on IVF success rates [6]; however, more objective clinical evidence is required before this can be implemented into practice worldwide.

2.2 Criteria to Trigger

Ensuring the correct timing of maturation trigger injections for oocyte retrieval is vital to achieve the best quality and number of oocytes following gonadotrophin stimulation. If oocytes are too small, then the likelihood is that they will be too immature for successful fertilisation. If the oocytes are too big, then, similarly, they may be post-mature and equally lead to poor fertilisation rates. It is therefore essential that trigger injections for final maturation are given at the correct point in follicular stimulation.

It is generally understood that follicles between 16 and 22 mm in diameter are more likely to yield mature oocytes, whereas those above or below these measurements lead to poorer-quality oocytes (on the day of oocyte retrieval). As follicles will grow approximately 1.7 mm/day, you would expect that the follicle size on the day of trigger may be 3–4 mm smaller than they would be on the day of retrieval [7]. In the study by Abbara et al., follicles that measured 12–19 mm on day of trigger made the greatest contribution to the number of oocytes retrieved [7]. They also suggested

that the sizes of follicles that contributed to the formation of embryos and high-quality embryos were comparable to those contributing to oocytes and mature oocytes.

It was also noted that when there is a higher ratio of follicles >17 mm:>10 mm, the chances of implantation, clinical pregnancy rate and live birth rate increased. Standard procedure is that once there are three or more follicles greater than 17 mm, then the trigger injection can be given.

Other criteria for determination of triggering can also be based on oestradiol levels; however, this is not routine in many clinics nowadays and is dependent on treatment centre preference. The trial by Hu et al. compared oestradiol with oocyte numbers and subsequent IVF success rates [8]. Mature ovum rate, fertilisation rate and good-quality embryo rate exhibited an increasing trend as the peak oestradiol level per oocyte increased, while pregnancy rate, implantation rate and live birth rate were found to be lower whenever the oestradiol:oocyte ratio exceeded 1,470 pmol/l per oocyte or was less than 370 pmol/l per oocyte [8].

Future determination of follicular maturity may be improved by the use of colour Doppler to detect vascularity of the ovarian stroma. Follicles that have more than 75% of their surface perfused, ovarian stromal peak systolic velocity of more than 10 cm/s and a resistance index of less than 0.4–0.48 have been shown to contain mature oocytes of satisfactory quality and result in a better grade of embryo. Follicles having a perifollicular blood flow of >50% have increased oocyte retrieval rates, with increased numbers of mature oocytes with higher fertilisation rates and lower triploidy rates, and lead to the formation of more higher-grade embryos [2]. The use of colour Doppler in the future has the potential for identification of better timing for final triggering of oocyte maturation; however, this has yet to be tested in comparison with mean follicle diameter, and further trials are needed to determine the effectiveness of this technique.

2.3 Timing between Trigger and Oocyte Retrieval

In a physiological state, LH surges will result in ovulation after 24–56 hours, with 32 hours being the mean time. However, during a COS cycle, there is an absence of natural endogenous LH surge. Therefore, an exogenous gonadotrophin is required to replace the natural LH surge, most commonly human chorionic gonadotropin (hCG). Determining the timing when this trigger injection needs to be given is crucial for the final stages of oocyte development and maturity, and is still a debated topic for the optimal time for triggering.

Initially, oocyte retrieval was to be performed within 36 hours of the trigger injection to minimise the risk of ovulation and loss of oocytes, based on the duration between LH surge and ovulation that occurs in the natural physiological process.

The interval between trigger injection and oocyte retrieval is important, because a series of crucial processes, such as the start of luteinisation, expansion of cumulus cells and the resumption of oocyte meiosis, are accomplished during this time. Therefore, if oocyte retrieval is performed too soon, the oocytes will be immature, while too late there is a risk of postmaturity and ovulation leading to the loss of oocytes.

A meta-analysis of previous studies by Wang et al. looked at five randomised controlled trials to determine the optimal time delay between trigger injection and oocyte retrieval [9]. Their conclusion was that there was no significant difference between fertilisation, implantation or pregnancy rates between those whose oocyte retrieval occurred before or after 36 hours from their trigger injection. Of note, there were more mature oocytes in metaphase II in patients whose trigger was more than 36 hours before their oocyte collection in comparison with those who had oocyte collection less than 36 hours from their trigger.

Spontaneous ovulation from prolonged exposure to trigger injection is still something to be mindful of. However, several studies have reported first follicular rupture/ovulation occurring anywhere from 38 to 41 hours after trigger injection [10].

Aiming for oocyte retrieval between 36 and 38 hours after trigger injection would be the ideal target to ensure more mature oocytes while not risking follicular rupture and ovulation and potential cancellation of treatment cycles.

2.4 Type of Trigger Injection

In the normal menstrual cycle, the final maturation of the oocyte occurs with a surge in LH and to a smaller degree FSH. In IVF, the need to mimic this physiological process is essential to develop metaphase II oocytes that will subsequently be mature enough to inseminated and create embryos.

However, simply using recombinant LH to do this has proven not to be an effective method. LH administration has been thoroughly reviewed over the years and been found to be an inferior method for triggering final maturation of oocytes in COS cycles. Instead, hCG is used predominately as the triggering agent. hCG is very similar structurally to LH, and both of them act on the same receptor, eliciting similar but not identical physiological responses.

In comparison, hCG has a significantly longer half-life than LH, 2–3 days compared with 1–5 hours, respectively, with hCG also being five times more potent. The reduced half-life and potency of LH limits its duration of effect and consequently the maturation of oocytes. A multicentre study of LH administration versus hCG for final oocyte maturation found that there were similar success rates between the two groups [11]. However, much higher doses of LH (15,000–30,000 IU) were required for similar success rates compared with the hCG group (5,000 IU), raising serious cost versus efficacy concerns. A subsequent Cochrane review also found the evidence regarding LH performance to be very low, which strongly limits the ability to draw any conclusions regarding its use for triggering, even when ignoring cost issues [12].

The doses of hCG trigger injections range from 1,500 to 15,000 IU, with the most common dose being 5,000 or 10,000 IU. Abdalla et al. showed that doses of 2,000 IU in comparison with 5,000 or 10,000 IU had a reduced oocyte recovery rate, with no significant difference between the 5,000 and 10,000 IU dose [13]. An increase in pregnancy rates was not confirmed with higher doses of hCG [14]. With increased doses of hCG up to 10,000 or 15,000 IU, there was no difference in oocyte yield in comparison with a dose of 5,000 IU [14]. Patients with a raised body mass index (BMI) do have lower levels of circulating hCG following the trigger shot, but a study by Hoyos et al. showed no difference in clinical pregnancy rate with standard hCG dose irrespective of BMI [15]. When increasing the dose, however, this also increases the risk of OHSS, and patients who received 5,000 IU were less likely to develop OHSS in comparison with the 10,000 IU group.

The use of either recombinant or urinary preparations of hCG has also been debated. Historically, urinary hCG has been the sole preparation used, but there were questions with regard to variation in hormone levels, potential transmission of disease and antibody formation. The ability to create recombinant hCG preparations has led to higher purity and a better safety profile in comparison with urinary hCG-based preparations, albeit at a greater production cost. This raised the question as to which would perform better clinically, with the result being that neither medication was significantly superior to the other.

The main issue of using hCG triggers is the risk of OHSS. hCG is considered important in OHSS due to its ability to upregulate vascular endothelial growth factor expression in granulosa cells, driving the hyperpermeability that causes OHSS to develop. In previous long cycles of stimulation, this was the only trigger injection that could be used, and in those who over-responded there was no option but to still trigger them with hCG, coast until the oestradiol levels fell or cancel the cycle. Introduction of the short GnRH antagonist cycle for stimulation has allowed the use of a GnRH agonist (GnRH-a) as a trigger for final oocyte maturation. Doses for GnRH-a triggers tend to be 0.5–2 mg for buserelin, 0.1–0.3 mg for triptorelin and 0.5–4 mg for leuprolide acetate. There has been no conclusive evidence that increasing the dose of the GnRH-a trigger improves outcomes with regard to oocyte numbers or maturity, although occasionally (in 1–2%) no eggs may be retrieved with lower doses. In this situation, it is recommended to stop collection after the first ovary, administer either 1,500 or 5,000 IU hCG depending on OHSS concerns, and collect from the second ovary 36 hours later.

GnRH-a significantly reduces the risk of OHSS, with the likelihood of patients developing moderate or severe OHSS being between 0% and 3% for a GnRH trigger in comparison with a 5% risk in those with an hCG trigger [16]. There is no difference in oocyte maturity, fertilisation rates or embryo development between hCG and GnRH-a triggers. However, the use of GnRH-a alone reduces the live birth rate, while increasing the risk of miscarriage. This is due to the lack of luteal support provided with a GnRH-a trigger compared with an hCG trigger, which has been attributed to the shorter half-life of the GnRH-a. Therefore, the use of a GnRH trigger alone should be reserved for those at risk of OHSS or those with planned elective freeze alls, such as those undergoing fertility preservation or oocyte donation.

Recently, there has been development of a 'dual-trigger' mechanism to achieve final oocyte maturation. The aim of this is to achieve decent oocyte maturation, embryo development and luteal support while reducing the risk of developing OHSS. A dual trigger means that GnRH-a and low-dose hCG (1,500 IU) are given at the same time and oocyte collection occurs 36 hours later. Recently, there have been promising results with administration of a dual trigger, but more research is required to determine its efficacy. There appear to be higher pregnancy rates with the dual triggers compared with GnRH triggers alone, but there is a higher chance of OHSS, although it is not as high as in those receiving a standard dose of hCG [17]. Luteal support during these studies was the same in both groups, and progesterone and oestrogen levels were monitored and doses of support were adjusted accordingly. There was no difference between the two groups in terms of their hormonal profile following dual or single trigger, despite being on the same luteal support.

Kisspeptin is another new trigger that has been developed recently. Kisspeptins are a group of hypothalamic arginine–phenylalanine amide peptides and act at the kisspeptin receptor on GnRH neurons in the hypothalamus to elicit endogenous GnRH release [14]. There have been a number of trials looking into the effect of kisspeptin and the dosing required. One of the first studies by Jayasena et al. showed that a single dose of kisspeptin given 36 hours prior to oocyte retrieval showed a dose-dependent mature oocyte yield (percentage of mature oocytes from follicles >14 mm on day of kisspeptin administration), with 36–49% at 1.6–3.2 nmol/kg, 76% at 6.4 nmol/kg and 103% at 12.8 nmol/kg [18]. The live birth rate per protocol was 19%. A subsequent study reviewed the benefit of an additional dose of kisspeptin 10 hours after the initial dose [14]. This increased the live birth rate to 39% in comparison with the single-dose group, whose live birth rate was 19%. Kisspeptin has also been used with patients at risk of OHSS. The study by Abbara et al. reviewed 60 women at risk of OHSS; only three developed mild OHSS, with none of them developing moderate to severe OHSS [14]. Kisspeptin is still new to assisted reproductive technology treatments, and further studies and comparisons with current ovulation triggers are required to determine its effectiveness and future role in reproductive medicine.

The serum profiles over time of the various triggers discussed are shown in Figure 2.1.

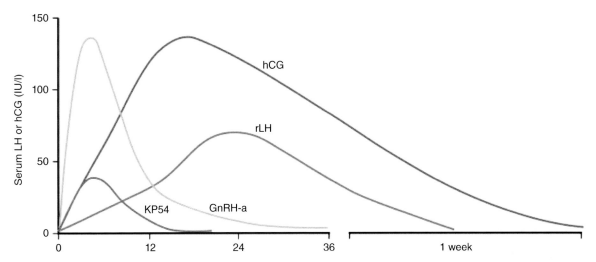

Figure 2.1 Serum profiles of inductors of oocyte maturation. The *x*-axis shows time (hours) after administration. hCG, human chorionic gonadotropin; rLH, recombinant luteinising hormone; GnRH-a, gonadotropin-releasing hormone antagonist; KP54, kisspeptin-54. A black and white version of this figure will appear in some formats. For the colour version, refer to the plate section. Reproduced from Abbara et al. [14].

2.5 Pre-operative Assessment for Oocyte Retrieval

Most oocyte retrievals are done using intravenous sedation, with a transvaginal approach being the most common. The benefit of sedation is that it is quick to administer, short acting, provides good analgesia and is associated with a good recovery profile. The transvaginal route is also the least invasive and traumatic approach to retrieve oocytes for the majority of IVF patients.

However, these approaches are not suitable for all patients, and good pre-operative assessment is essential in all patients about to undergo oocyte retrieval to ensure patient safety throughout the IVF process.

Understanding the capabilities of your specific unit is also necessary to determine whether you can take higher-risk patients and deal with them safely. Pre-operative assessment will help identify equipment, facilities and staffing capabilities required for more complex oocyte retrievals and aims to prevent procedures being performed in a setting that is unsuitable and unsafe for certain patients.

Most patients undergoing oocyte retrievals are women between 20 and 40 years of age. As a group, they tend to be relatively healthy, but consideration must be taken to review their past medical history. Causes for their subfertility such as raised BMI, cystic fibrosis, fibroids and endometriosis all have an impact on how you approach the oocyte retrieval. This

approach needs to be considered particularly in those with raised BMI or multiple fibroids, and the transvaginal approach may not be the optimum route; therefore, an abdominal or laparoscopic approach may be necessary. Those with airway issues due to comorbidities such as raised BMI, poorly controlled asthma or cystic fibrosis may also require an anaesthetic review prior to retrieval to determine the anaesthetic technique required to ensure the best outcome for the patient. The above can all be determined at the pre-operative assessment and can allow appropriate planning prior to the procedure.

This is a group of patients who are at increased risk of venous thromboembolism, although the mechanism for this is unknown. One theory is that high oestrogen levels associated with ovarian stimulation may induce a pro-coagulant effect by increasing levels of coagulation factors such as von Willebrand factor, factor VIII, factor V and fibrinogen, while decreasing levels of the anticoagulants protein S and antithrombin. While ovulation induction itself is not an indication on its own to initiate thromboprophylaxis, if coupled with other risks factors, then low-molecular-weight heparin may be indicated.

2.6 Consent

When preparing a patient for any procedure, informed consent must be obtained. This allows them to make a decision fully knowing the risks and complications of a procedure and consequently granting permission for it to take place.

Oocyte retrieval in the majority of cases is a low-risk procedure but the known complications are listed below:

- Infection. Following needle insertion, bacteria that were present in the vagina may be passed into the abdominal cavity. The estimated incidence of bacterial infection is less than 0.5% [19] and can affect the uterus, Fallopian tubes, ovaries or other abdominal organs. The use of antibiotics for this procedure is not routine, but those who may be at risk, such as those with endometriomas or if the aspiration needle has passed close to or been in contact with bowel, would be candidates for prophylaxis.
- Bleeding. Small amounts of bleeding are common with oocyte retrieval, occurring in 8–25% of cases. This is to be expected with multiple blood vessels adjacent to the needle insertion point, as well as the roof of the vagina and ovary. The incidence of major bleeding is estimated to be less than 0.1%.
- Trauma. Insertion of the aspiration needle into the abdominal cavity has the potential to cause damage to the surrounding structures, including the bowel, bladder, ureters and blood vessels. If significant damage is caused, then further surgery may be indicated; however, this might not be identified until patients reattend when they are unwell. Nurse triage sheets are important to document patient callbacks and to identify the sick patient.
- Anaesthesia risks (see Chapter 4).
- Failure. This comes in multiple forms. It may be that despite aspiration of a follicle, no oocytes are retrieved, or fewer oocytes are retrieved than anticipated. Some ovaries may be inaccessible at the time of oocyte retrieval. The potential of failed implantation or pregnancy also needs to be discussed with the patient.

- Pain. Mild pain is to be expected following this procedure. Simple analgesia should suffice; however, some patients may experience more pain than others and may need stronger pain relief. Some may need further investigating if potential damage to intra-abdominal organs is a concern. Post-oocyte retrieval pain can sometimes be difficult to differentiate from OHSS symptoms. A haematocrit is the best marker, being raised in the haemoconcentrated state of OHSS.

2.7 Summary

Monitoring of ovarian stimulation is a complex and ever-changing process that is under constant review. Our aims remains the same – ensuring good oocyte numbers and maturity, avoiding OHSS and, above all, improving pregnancy and live birth rates.

Confirming appropriate follicular growth on ultrasound will enable the identification of when to trigger patients and also identify those at risk of OHSS. Ultrasound enables clinicians to ensure that no other pathologies are present prior to stimulation and allows intervention if required to reduce any potential impact of COS cycles. Advances in ultrasound with regard to Doppler flow and 3D imaging are exciting prospects for improving our understanding of the ovarian stimulation cycle.

The use of hormonal monitoring throughout treatment is less intensive than before, with the use of oestradiol monitoring adding little to the determination of trigger when ultrasound measurements on their own can determine this. However, a better understanding of hormonal profiles, such as the early progesterone rise, may help to determine those in need of intervention or cycle adjustment to improve their treatment outcomes.

Better future understanding of dual triggers, or kisspeptin for final oocyte maturation, may lead to improvements in pregnancy rates and a further reduction of moderate to severe OHSS.

References

1. Hardiman P, Thomas M, Osgood V, Vlassopoulou V, Ginsburg J. (1990) Are estrogen assays essential for monitoring gonadotropin stimulant therapy? *Gynecol Endocrinol* 4(4):261–9. doi: 10.3109/09513599009024980

2. Patil M. Monitoring ovarian stimulation: current perspectives. In: Allahbadia GN, Morimoto Y, eds. *Ovarian Stimulation Protocols*. New Delhi: Springer, 2016; 17–55.

3. Salama S., Torre A, Paillusson B, et al. Ovarian stimulation

monitoring: past, present and perspectives. *Gynecol Obstet Fertil* 2011;39(4):245–54. doi: 10.1016/j. gyobfe.2011.02.003

4. Ryan A, Wang S, Alvero R, Polotsky AJ. Prolonged gonadotropin stimulation for assisted reproductive technology

cycles is associated with decreased pregnancy rates for all women except for women with polycystic ovary syndrome. *J Assist Reprod Genet* 2014;**31**(7):837–42. doi: 10.1007/s10815-014-0253-9

5. Kwan I, Bhattacharya S, Kang A, Woolner A. Monitoring of stimulated cycles in assisted reproduction (IVF and ICSI). *Cochrane Database Syst Rev* 2014;**8**:CD005289. doi: 10.1002/14651858.CD005289.pub3

6. Lawrenz B, Labarta E, Fatemi H, Bosch E. Premature progesterone elevation: targets and rescue strategies. *Fertil Steril* 2018;**109**(4):577–82. doi: 10.1016/j.fertnstert.2018.02.128

7. Abbara A, Vuong LN, Ho VNA, et al. Follicle size on day of trigger most likely to yield a mature oocyte. *Front Endocrinol (Lausanne)* 2018;**9**:193. doi:10.3389/fendo.2018.00193

8. Hu X, Luo Y, Huang K, et al. New perspectives on criteria for the determination of HCG trigger timing in GnRH antagonist cycles. *Medicine (Baltimore)* 2016;**95**(20):e3691. doi: 10.1097/MD.0000000000003691

9. Wang W, Zhang XH, Wang WH, et al. The time interval between hCG priming and oocyte retrieval in ART program: a meta-analysis. *J Assist Reprod Genet* 2011;**28**(10):901–10. doi: 10.1007/s10815-011-9613-x

10. Andersen AG, Als-Nielsen B, Hornnes PJ, Franch Andersen L. Time interval from human chorionic gonadotrophin (HCG) injection to follicular rupture. *Hum Reprod* 1995;**10**(12):3202–5. doi: 10.1093/oxfordjournals.humrep.a135888

11. European Recombinant LH Study Group. Human recombinant luteinizing hormone is as effective as, but safer than, urinary human chorionic gonadotropin in inducing final follicular maturation and ovulation in in vitro fertilization procedures: results of a multicenter double-blind study. *J Clin Endocrinol Metab* 2001;**86**(6):2607–18. doi: 10.1210/jcem.86.6.7599

12. Youssef MA, Abou-Setta AM, Lam WS. Recombinant versus urinary human chorionic gonadotrophin for final oocyte maturation triggering in IVF and ICSI cycles. *Cochrane Database Syst Rev* 2016;**4**:CD003719. doi: 10.1002/14651858.CD003719.pub4

13. Abdalla HI, Ah-Moye M, Brinsden P, et al. The effect of the dose of human chorionic gonadotropin and the type of gonadotropin stimulation on oocyte recovery rates in an in vitro fertilization program. *Fertil Steril* 1987;**48**(6):958–63. doi: 10.1016/s0015-0282(16)59591-0

14. Abbara A, Clarke SA, Dhillo WS. Novel concepts for inducing final oocyte maturation in in vitro fertilization treatment. *Endocr Rev* 2018;**39**(5):593628. doi: 10.1210/er.2017-00236

15. Hoyos LR, Khan S, Dai J, et al. Low-dose urinary human chorionic gonadotropin is effective for oocyte maturation in in vitro fertilization/intracytoplasmic sperm injection cycles independent of body mass index. *Int J Fertil Steril* 2016;**11**(1):7–14. doi: 10.22074/ijfs.2016.5145

16. Youssef MAFM, van der Veen F, Al-Inany HG, et al. Gonadotropin-releasing hormone agonist versus HCG for oocyte triggering in antagonist-assisted reproductive technology. *Cochrane Database Syst Rev* 2014;**10**:CD008046. doi: 10.1002/14651858.CD008046.pub4

17. Engmann LL, Maslow BS, Kaye LA, et al. Low dose human chorionic gonadotropin administration at the time of gonadotropin releasing-hormone agonist trigger versus 35 h later in women at high risk of developing ovarian hyperstimulation syndrome – a prospective randomized double-blind clinical trial. *J Ovarian Res* 2019;**12**(1):8. doi: 10.1186/s13048-019-0483-7

18. Jayasena CN, Abbara A, Comninos AN, et al. Kisspeptin-54 triggers egg maturation in women undergoing in vitro fertilization. *J Clin Invest* 2014;**124**(8): 3667–77. doi: 10.1172/JCI75730

19. Govaerts I, Devreker F, Delbaere A, Revelard P, Englert Y. Short-term medical complications of 1500 oocyte retrievals for in vitro fertilization and embryo transfer. *Eur J Obstet Gynecol Reprod Biol* 1998;**77**(2):239–43. doi: 10.1016/s0301-2115(97)00263-7

Theatre Design, Equipment and Consumables for Oocyte Retrieval

Lukasz Polanski and Alka Prakash

3.1 Introduction

The theatre space is integral to an in vitro fertilisation (IVF) unit. This is where key steps of IVF such as oocyte retrieval and embryo transfer are performed. Hence, it is critical that we optimise this to ensure patient safety and facilitate better success rates. Another key point to consider while organising the process flow around oocyte collection is to future proof with a view to accommodating further developments that happen in the assisted conception unit at a later date. In this chapter, we will discuss the concepts that need to be considered when designing a theatre and the basic equipment required to provide quality care for the patients. Busy IVF centres rely on a rapid changeover of patients, and efficient design of the admissions lounge, theatre and recovery space aids in efficiency and increases the throughput of patients without compromising their care.

3.2 Design Considerations

In simple terms, the theatre utilised for oocyte collection should comfortably accommodate the teams that will be using it to provide a safe environment for the patient and staff. As such, the physical space should be large enough to accommodate a wash basin/sink, operating bed, anaesthetic machine, ultrasound machine, oocyte aspiration instruments, medicine cupboards, emergency medications and equipment, and easy access to the laboratory section. It should be well lit with adequate air exchange. Each of these items will be discussed below.

When considering the patient journey through the fertility clinic on the day of oocyte collection, each step should be made as stress free for the patient as possible. This is a day that will influence the realistic chance of conception and, as such, is perceived as a 'make or break' moment by many infertile couples. Additional stress may be perceived as a cause for an unsuccessful cycle. After entering the clinic, the patients are sat in the waiting area, following which they are taken to the recovery space or admissions lounge. This allows the patient to be seen by the operator and anaesthetist in a quiet space before oocyte collection. This space would usually be comprised of cubicles with curtain dividers or, in larger units, separate rooms with adequate sound insulation. This allows privacy when discussing the upcoming procedure and any confidential details that the patient wishes to disclose to the operator or anaesthetist. Having an open recovery area allows easy oversight of many patients at the same time by a limited number of nursing staff but may be perceived as lacking confidentiality by patients due to the lack of physical walls. Where central monitoring systems are in place, or there are sufficient staff dedicated to recover patients after the procedure, individual rooms would be an appropriate option. Each bed space should, however, permit 360-degree access to the patient and have electric sockets, access to medical gas, a dimmable light and an emergency button. In line with the *Health Building Note (HBN) 26: Facilities for surgical procedures: Volume 1*, the recovery area as well as the theatre should have access to natural daylight [1]. For recovery, this is true; however, for the purposes of oocyte collection, exposure to any light should be minimised to limit the possible damage to the oocyte [2].

When designing the theatre space with associated facilities, infection control issues need to be considered, with easy access to every surface and use of non-porous materials that are easy to clean. Accessible facilities for the handicapped should also be borne in mind when organising the procedure room. Due to the nature of IVF units, single-sex facilities are the standard, with the exception of the need for occasional surgical sperm retrieval, where the man could be located in a separate bay or recovery room. The recovery/admissions lounge areas should have easy and sufficient access to bathroom facilities, as, prior to oocyte retrieval, the patient is asked to empty their bladder to allow better visualisation of pelvic organs and minimise the risk of damage to the distended bladder. Similarly, stress before the procedure increases the frequency of urination in many patients. Following assessment by the medical team, the patient is taken into the operating theatre. It is important that the route is not too long and does not lead through a cold corridor or public access spaces, as at this point hospital gowns are what most patients would be wearing. The siting of the theatre should be considered at the initial stages of a new building, and in case of adaptation of existing buildings, the theatre, recovery and admissions lounge spaces should be located centrally within the organisation, in proximity to each other. In stand-alone units, an easy route to move the patient on the bed and out of the building in an emergency should be envisaged, with easy access to lifts in a multistorey building. In units embedded within hospitals, access to critical care services should be direct, and easy access to emergency care, imaging services and the anaesthetic department should be possible with minimal effort [1]. A necessary requirement for procedure room location within the IVF unit is the direct proximity to the laboratory for quick and easy transfer of oocytes and embryos. Staff changing facilities should also be located in the vicinity to minimise the exposure of scrubs to possible outside contaminants [3].

3.3 Anaesthetic Room

If an anaesthetic room is present, this should be at least 19 m^2 and able to accommodate the patient on the bed and at least four people with additional anaesthetic equipment. A ceiling-mounted, adjustable lamp should be present. A lockable controlled-drugs cabinet with a medicines fridge should be within easy reach [1]. Hand-washing facilities with non-touch controls should be present.

3.4 Procedure Room

In line with National Health Service guidance, all theatres for minimal invasive surgery should be at least 55 m^2 with a 3 m floor-to-ceiling clearance [1]. This may be a luxury for small units where space is at a premium; however 42 m^2 is the minimal recommendation by International Health Facility

Guidelines and refers specifically to oocyte retrieval rooms. Access to electric sockets and medical gas should be unobstructed. A dedicated work bench for a computer should be present in order to retrieve medical information, especially now due to the drive for paperless health records. A working phone line with the ability to dial internal and external contacts is recommended [1, 3].

In theatre, the patient is greeted by the staff, who should include as a minimum an anaesthetist, an anaesthetic assistant, the person performing the oocyte collection and an assistant. The operating table should be modifiable to the need of the procedure, sturdy enough to assure stability and mobile enough to change its position easily. The options include a non-removable operating table, or a mobile trolley that is versatile enough to be used as an operating table and recovery bed. The latter has the advantage of wheeling the patient out of theatre on the bed without the need for transfer from the operating table onto the recovery bed. This will require a significant number of such beds, which may increase the overall costs of running the unit. Equipment to lift and turn the unconscious patient should be present, as there may be need for its use irrespective of what type operating beds are used [1]. The decision as to which beds to use will depend on the numbers of patients treated, as well as the unit's financial situation. In either case, the bottom half of the operating bed/table needs to flex or be removable in order to gain vaginal access. Robust stirrups need to be fitted securely to the sides of the bed. The bed should be positioned in the middle of the theatre space with sufficient ceiling-mounted lighting that can be angled to allow good visibility of the cervix. The theatre light should also be able to dim or switch off completely with unobstructed access to the controls.

Positioning of the patient is important, and it is preferable to assure it is done appropriately while the patient is still awake. The patient is asked to sit on the edge of the bed in between the stirrups (with the bottom half of the bed removed) or lie on the bed with the buttocks level with the break in the bed (at the junction of the fixed and mobile parts of the operating table). Practices vary, but it is acceptable to ask the patient to place her legs in stirrups assuring dignity, especially if the oocyte collection is done under local anaesthetic, or to position the patient's legs in the supports once the patient is under sedation. It is important to have easy access to the patient from all sides and to be able to accommodate more staff if an emergency arises. A wall-mounted emergency button should be present in the theatre in a easily visible and accessible location. An emergency trolley with a defibrillator should be present on the theatre premises or in the immediate vicinity [1].

Once the patient is positioned appropriately, which includes the buttocks being on the edge of the bed with the legs safety supported by the stirrups, the additional equipment should be positioned close to the patient. This includes the ultrasound machine used for oocyte retrieval, aspiration equipment, oocyte collection tube warmer and chair for the person performing the procedure. Similarly as in the anaesthetic room, adequate hand-washing facilities with non-touch taps should be within the oocyte retrieval room or in a separate, adjoining scrub area. In the absence of the latter, a dedicated area to lay out open sterile gowns or gloves should be available. In the aforementioned HNB 26 document, examples of theatre layout and adjoining facilities are presented, but these are mainly dedicated to major surgical cases, and as such should only be treated as guidance for designing oocyte collection theatres [1].

Conventionally, the ultrasound machine is positioned on the right side of the patient; however, this may vary depending on the user, as well as the theatre layout. The operator sits in between the patient's legs on a mobile stool. Preparation of the operating field commences once the patient is anaesthetised. Cleaning of the perineum and vagina prior to oocyte retrieval is standard practice. This should be done with solutions that are non-toxic to oocytes and do not cause significant mucous membrane irritation. Most commonly this is normal saline, as the use of 0.5% chlorhexidine solutions or povidone iodine has not been shown to be superior in minimising the risk of infection following oocyte retrieval and have the potential to damage oocytes [4, 5]. A transvaginal scan is performed to orientate the operator and assess the pelvic organs before oocyte retrieval, following which the oocyte aspiration needle is introduced through the needle guide. The vaginal puncture area should be selected based on the proximity to the ovary (only the vaginal wall and peritoneum) and absence of blood vessels that could be injured. When such direct access is not possible, pressure by the assistant on the abdomen may bring the ovary lower into the pelvis or stabilise it enough to assure safe access. Occasionally, transmyometrial or transabdominal access may be needed. This should be carried out by experienced operators, and antibiotic prophylaxis should be considered in line with local policies and antibiotic resistance [6].

The length of tubing connecting the needle to the suction equipment is a limiting factor in the positioning of the equipment. The equipment should be close enough to the operator not to restrict their movements during oocyte collection and to avoid bending the tubing, which may damage the oocytes and reduce suction pressure, and to avoid inadvertent pulling on the line when changing tubes, which may lead to pelvic organ injury. Placement of the patient just at the edge of the bed, or even slightly off it, allows easy access to the ovaries, even if they are very anteriorly positioned. Changing the position of the patient when the needle has been inserted may lead to organ damage or increase the risk of infection with multiple vaginal wall punctures.

The tube with follicular fluid is then passed to the laboratory for assessment. This should be done as soon as possible, as any cooling of the tube or unnecessary light exposure may affect the success rates of the clinic. Data on the direct effect of light exposure and damage to the oocyte and embryo are limited in humans; however, animal studies have shown a detrimental developmental effect. Light wavelengths of less than 500 nm (blue visible and ultraviolet light) seem to be the most damaging [2]. Hence, it is important to be able to block out natural light in the operating theatre and/or work stations where gametes and embryos are handled. All light should be dimmed for the duration of the procedure. The use of green bypass filters may also decrease the exposure to potentially harmful light while not compromising the ability to assess embryo development [7]. A runner may be utilised if the distance to the laboratory is significant, or the assistant places the tube in a hatch with another tube warmer. Cooling of the oocytes below 35°C leads to depolymerisation of the meiotic spindle and damage to the oocyte. The spindle may reassemble when temperature rises; however, incorrect reassembly may lead to non-disjunction events causing aneuploidy [8]. The biggest factor that cools the tubing is high air flow. Hence, the procedure of oocyte collection should be carried out as quickly as possible and passage of the samples done as efficiently as is feasible [9]. At the end of the procedure, the needle and tubing need to be disposed of safely, and easy and close access to large sharps bins is essential to minimise any risks of injury or spillage. After the procedure is complete, a careful inspection of the vaginal walls is essential to assure that there is no significant bleeding, which should be tackled with pressure or appropriate stitches. A mobile, overhead operating light is essential at this point to aid in such assessment.

3.5 Air Quality

Air quality in the oocyte collection room should be as good as possible and the routine use of high-efficiency particulate air (HEPA) filters may aid this requirement. Where patient skin is exposed, the air quality is unlikely to be better than grade D (up to 120 colony-forming units (CFU)/m^3) unless laminar flow hoods are in routine operation. Daily cleaning of the procedure room and deep cleaning sessions should be scheduled in line with local policies. All theatre staff should therefore wear protective clothing (scrubs) and a hat to attempt to improve the air quality within the theatre room. Air quality in the laboratory areas should be of much better purity. In order to ensure as little microbial contamination as possible within the actual laboratory where gametes and embryos are handled (grade A or B at least; <1 CFU/m^3 and 10 CFU/m^3, respectively), hermetically sealed pass-throughs between the areas of procurement of gametes and the clean laboratory should be in place [9].

3.6 Equipment

When considering equipment that is necessary to operate an IVF centre, one should consider the patient flow from the admissions lounge through the procedure room to recovery. On admission, a set of observations needs to be taken, which includes blood pressure readings, pulse rate and oxygen saturation as a minimum. This requires either manual or automated devices capable of carrying out these readings accurately. Each unit must therefore have a procedure for procuring and assuring the accuracy of such devices by regular quality and safety checks. In theatre, the most essential piece of equipment is the anaesthetic machine. This assures the patient's safety while under sedation for the oocyte collection. Modern anaesthetic machines are capable of keeping the majority of patients safely sedated with minimal input from the operator, but the presence of an anaesthetist is mandatory. Continuous non-invasive

monitoring of blood pressure, pulse, oxygen saturation and electrocardiogram (ECG) readings are the minimal standards for safe anaesthesia [10]. An oxygen mask with tubing should be applied in every case and should be readily available. Intubation equipment, although rarely needed, should be present in case of emergency. Medicine cabinets and fridges have been already mentioned and should be within easy reach of the anaesthetist or their assistant. These cabinets should be restocked on a regular basis with stocks updated according to the use and expiry date of medications. Procurement of anaesthetic equipment should be carried out following discussion with the anaesthetic department, as they will be able to assess directly whether the equipment meets the needs of the unit and is sufficient for the capacity. An anaesthetic machine should have continuous access to medical gases and vacuum.

An ultrasound machine is the next most essential piece of equipment that is required. The machine should be mobile and equipped with high-frequency transvaginal and transabdominal transducers in order to be able to carry out oocyte collection via the vaginal and abdominal routes and aid in guiding embryo transfers. Most modern ultrasound machines are capable of a wide range of settings, but, as a minimum, these should include gain and depth adjustment, focal zone toggles and Doppler capabilities, and it should display the superimposed needle guide. A compatible probe-mounted needle guide is required, which clips onto the transducer and allows controlled introduction of the oocyte aspiration needle and assures a steady path along the displayed needle guide. A sterile, powder-free, non-latex probe cover should be used with good-quality sterile coupling gel to ensure good and uninterrupted vision throughout the procedure.

A sharp, 17–18-gauge needle is most commonly used, as it has been shown to reduce discomfort and minimise damage to the oocytes and ovaries, while at the same time ensuring a good oocyte harvest [11]. Lancet-shaped, bevelled needles are recommended, as they are easy to see on ultrasound and the design helps to localise the tip easily. The attached tubing should be translucent to allow the operator to see the aspirated fluid. Some units use larger, double-lumen needles that allow flushing of the follicles in order to obtain more oocytes, especially in poor responders. A systematic review of the literature has suggested that such practice has little or no effect on live births (odds ratio

0.95; 95% confidence interval 0.58–1.56), and also does not significantly improve the oocyte yield, total embryo number or number of cryopreserved embryos [12].

A suction pump attached to the needle via the tubing generates the necessary negative pressure to allow aspiration of the follicles. A steady pressure should be maintained throughout the procedure, unless a blockage is encountered. The evidence does not seem to suggest one safe pressure level, provided the device operates within the manufacturer's recommended parameters. A pressure in excess of 200 mmHg should not be used; however, high pressures of more than 140 mmHg have not been associated with damage to the oocyte. The most common setting ranges between 120 and 140 mmHg [13]. Every piece of equipment that comes in contact with the oocyte should have been tested and its embryo toxicity excluded. When purchasing such equipment, this should have been considered, with appropriate quality marks verified. The tubes that the follicular fluid is aspirated into should be pre-warmed in an appropriate warmer to a temperature of 36.4–36.9°C, as this assures optimal outcomes of treatment with the highest live birth rates compared with lower or higher temperatures (52.8% versus 44.1% and 37.7%, respectively; $P<0.05$) [14], with the Association of Clinical Embryologists recommending a steady temperature of 37°C [15]. This should be continuously checked with an appropriate thermometer. Deviation from this temperature should be quickly recognised and rectified.

3.7 Summary

Design of the 'heart and lungs' of the IVF unit requires forward planning, as all areas and fittings should be in place before the mobile equipment is introduced. Any omissions in the design and construction of the theatre and adjoining areas will result in costly reconstructions or will interrupt patient or gamete flow, resulting in patient distress, reduced success rates and, possibly, failure of the institution. A thought-out layout will maximise staff utilisation, with the ability to easily and quickly carry out procedures in adjacent theatres even by one practitioner (i.e. oocyte collection in one procedure room, embryo transfer in the next). The design of the admissions lounge, theatre, recovery space and laboratory should take into account the possibility of expansion, as each clinic aims to increase their numbers over time. Construction of such an expensive unit for current needs without future planning will restrict expansion and necessitate a change of premises or costly building additions, putting the running of the clinic on hold or significantly limiting ongoing patient care. The ultimate goal of the centre is to allow the patient to feel as relaxed and safe as possible during this stressful time, aiming for the highest live birth rates achievable. This includes a welcoming environment with natural daylight, background music, easy access to toilet facilities and privacy at all stages of the process, as well as helpful and understanding staff with excellent laboratory support.

It would be advisable to consult the relevant personnel at the design stages of a new purpose-built unit, as their insights into patient flow may be invaluable. In IVF, every efficiency may translate to a small increase in success rates, which in turn translates into significant gains for our patients.

References

1. NHS Estates. *HBN 26: Facilities for Surgical Procedures: Volume 1.* 2004. Available from: www.england.nhs.uk/publication/facilities-for-surgical-procedures-in-acute-general-hospitals-hbn-26/

2. Ottosen LD, Hindkjaer J, Ingerslev J. Light exposure of the ovum and preimplantation embryo during ART procedures. *J Assist Reprod Genet* 2007;**24** (2–3):99–103. doi: 10.1007/s10815-006-9081-x

3. International Health Facility Guidelines. *Part B – Health Facility Briefing & Design 140 IVF Unit (Fertilisation Centres).* 2014. Available from: http://healthfacilityguidelines.com/Guidelines/ViewPDF/iHFG/iHFG_part_b_IVF_unit

4. Mangram AJ, Horan TC, Pearson ML, Silver LC, Jarvis WR. Guideline for prevention of surgical site infection, 1999. Hospital Infection Control Practices Advisory Committee. *Infect Control Hosp Epidemiol* 1999;**20**(4):250–78. doi: 10.1086/501620

5. Ludwig AK, Glawatz M, Griesinger G, Diedrich K, Ludwig M. Perioperative and postoperative complications of transvaginal ultrasound-guided oocyte retrieval: prospective study of >1000 oocyte retrievals. *Hum Reprod* 2006;**21**(12):3235–40. doi: 10.1093/humrep/del278

6. Aslam B, Wang W, Arshad MI, et al. Antibiotic resistance: a

rundown of a global crisis. *Infect Drug Resist* 2018;**11**:1645–58. doi: 10.2147/IDR.S173867

7. Pomeroy KO, Reed ML. The effect of light on embryos and embryo culture. *J Reprod Stem Cell Biotechnol* 2013;**3**(2): 46–54. doi: 10.1177/205891581200300203

8. Pickering SJ, Braude PR, Johnson MH, Cant A, Currie J. Transient cooling to room temperature can cause irreversible disruption of the meiotic spindle in the human oocyte. *Fertil Steril* 1990;**54**(1):102–8. doi: 10.1016/s0015-0282(16)53644-9

9. Mortimer D. A critical assessment of the impact of the European Union Tissues and Cells Directive (2004) on laboratory practices in assisted conception. *Reprod Biomed Online* 2005;**11**(2):162–76. doi: 10.1016/s1472-6483(10)60954-6

10. Checketts MR, Alladi R, Ferguson K, et al. Recommendations for standards of monitoring during anaesthesia and recovery 2015: Association of Anaesthetists of Great Britain and Ireland. *Anaesthesia* 2016;**71**(1):85–93. doi: 10.1111/anae.13316

11. Awonuga A, Waterstone J, Oyesanya O, et al. A prospective randomized study comparing needles of different diameters for transvaginal ultrasound-directed follicle aspiration. *Fertil Steril* 1996;**65**(1):109–13. doi: 10.1016/s0015-0282(16)58036-4

12. Georgiou EX, Melo P, Brown J, Granne IE. Follicular flushing during oocyte retrieval in assisted reproductive techniques. *Cochrane Database Syst Rev* 2018;**4**:CD004634. doi: 10.1002/14651858.CD004634.pub3

13. Kumaran A, Narayan PK, Pai PJ, et al. Oocyte retrieval at 140-

mmHg negative aspiration pressure: a promising alternative to flushing and aspiration in assisted reproduction in women with low ovarian reserve. *J Hum Reprod Sci*, 2015;**8**(2):98–102. doi: 10.4103/0974-1208.158617

14. Sherbahn R. Assessment of effect of follicular fluid temperature at egg retrieval on blastocyst development, implantation and live birth rates. *Fertil Steril* 2010. **94**(4):S69–9. doi: 10.1016/j.fertnstert.2010.07.267

15. Hughes C, Association of Clinical Embryologists. Association of clinical embryologists – guidelines on good practice in clinical embryology laboratories 2012. *Hum Fertil (Camb)*, 2012;**15**(4):174–89. doi: 10.3109/14647273.2012.747891.

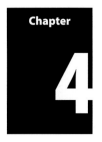

Conscious Sedation and Analgesia for Oocyte Retrieval

Jennifer M. Ulyatt and Sarah J. Martins da Silva

4.1 Introduction

Oocyte retrieval is a fundamental part of in vitro fertilisation (IVF). Various approaches are used to enable patient tolerance for this minor surgical procedure including general anaesthesia, conscious sedation and analgesia, deep sedation, patient-controlled analgesia and alternative therapies. However, a recent Cochrane review has suggested that none is superior in providing sedation and pain relief during and after oocyte retrieval [1].

Sedation describes a drug-induced depression of consciousness. There are three defined levels: anxiolysis, conscious sedation and deep sedation. For each level, there is an increasing depression of consciousness, associated airway vulnerability and depression of the cardiovascular system. Beyond this, general anaesthesia is a state of controlled unconsciousness where a patient is unable to safely support their airway, ventilation is often inadequate and airway reflexes are impaired [2].

Sedation and general anaesthesia lie on a continuum. However, sedation has a better recovery and safety profile than general anaesthesia and is therefore advantageous for day-case procedures. For this reason, it is an approach suited to oocyte retrieval. Indeed, conscious sedation and analgesia is the commonest approach used [3]. Conscious sedation requires the patient to maintain verbal communication. When responsiveness is reduced, the patient should still respond to vocal commands, either alone or with associated light tactile stimulation. No intervention should be required to maintain a patent airway, and spontaneous ventilation should always be adequate. However, because sedation is a continuum, it is not always possible to predict how an individual patient will respond. Of note, a deeper level of sedation has similar risks to general anaesthesia.

4.2 Pre-operative Assessment

Pre-operative assessment of all elective patients should be performed routinely prior to surgical procedures in line with recommendations of the Royal College of Anaesthetists [4]. Pre-operative assessment is a risk-assessment tool that highlights comorbidities that could adversely affect, or be affected by, sedation or anaesthesia. An integral part of the pre-operative assessment process is to take a full medical history, including documentation of current medication and any allergies. This allows planning and relevant intervention, including modification of drug therapies and consideration of potential drug interactions.

We recommend routine pre-assessment in preparation for oocyte retrieval. This provides personalised care but also offers the opportunity for health promotion, including weight, diet, benefits of exercise and smoking cessation, as well as ensuring prenatal folic acid and vitamin D supplements. This discussion is an important opportunity not only for preparation for fertility treatment and pregnancy but also for overall health and well-being [5]. It is worth noting that pre-assessment may occasionally identify patients who merit further medical assessment and investigation according to local policies and protocols, potentially resulting in a necessary delay in fertility treatment.

Another important feature of the pre-assessment process is the possibility of individualised support for fertility patients in preparation for treatment. Review by a member of the sedation team may be relevant for various reasons, including anxiety about sedation, phobias, a history of adverse events and/or other psychological issues. Pre-assessment allows patient preparation and personalised care by addressing specific concerns, and allows the opportunity to seek further medical information, investigation and/or specialist advice (if required), prior to oocyte retrieval. It may also involve counselling to support and prepare patients.

A pre-assessment clinic or PAC chart has been modified and developed for use in Ninewells Assisted Conception Unit (Dundee, UK) and is included as an example (Figure 4.1). It is simple for any healthcare practitioner to use and has a traffic-light system to highlight where there is a need for investigations or other concerns.

A further sedation consultation is performed on the day of egg retrieval, particularly to capture any changes in medical history, medications or allergies that may have occurred since pre-assessment [4]. It is important to use language that the patient under-stands, as good communication is vital to the patient's understanding of the sedation process as well as for building a relationship with the patient and relieving anxiety [6]. Patients often fear the unknown and have varied expectations regarding conscious sedation and oocyte retrieval. They may need reassurance that con-scious sedation, with titrated pain relief, is appropri-ate and will be effective. It is also important that the knowledge, skill and expertise of the clinician is relayed to the patient, as this will add to their reassurance [7].

4.3 Fasting Guidelines

Patients receiving any form of sedation or anaesthesia must follow fasting guidelines. Specifically, they should not eat for at least 6 hours and should have nothing to drink for at least 2 hours prior to sedation or anaesthetic [8]. This is to reduce the risk of aspir-ation of stomach contents (and potential death) in the absence of airway reflexes. On a practical note, if egg retrieval is in the morning, we advise fasting from midnight. Consumption of clear fluid (water, apple juice, tea or coffee with only a teaspoon of milk) is actively encouraged up until 2 hours prior to oocyte retrieval, and we alter this time depending on the time of theatre. It is also worth noting that a well-hydrated patient can reduce the risk of cardiovascular com-promise and make cannulation for intravenous (IV) access easier.

Diabetic patients need specific guidance regarding fasting and insulin or hypoglycaemic medication. Each hospital or fertility clinic should have clinical guidelines to cover this, which is outside the scope of this chapter. However, these patients are best placed first on a procedure list to avoid prolonged fasting

times, and it is essential to regularly monitor their blood sugars and act accordingly.

4.4 Sedation and Analgesia Medication for Oocyte Retrieval

Conscious sedation and analgesia are an effective combination to achieve pain-free oocyte retrieval. This is a safe approach in healthy individuals and has no known adverse effects on oocyte (or embryo) quality and/or pregnancy rates [3].

4.4.1 Midazolam

Midazolam is a short-acting benzodiazepine com-monly used for fertility procedures due to its sedative and anxiolytic effects [3]. Midazolam is also useful for its amnesic effect, although it is worth noting that benzodiazepines offer only anterograde amnesia, so it is important to ensure that they are given early or pre-procedure. Midazolam is unique from others in its drug class due to its rapid onset of effect (within 2 minutes) and short duration of action (half-life 1.5–2.5 hours), which allows quick recovery post-procedure.

Benzodiazepine drugs can have a depressant effect on the respiratory and cardiovascular system, although midazolam is thought to be less depressant than others in its class [9]. However, concurrent use of midazolam and opioids can increase the risk of apnoea and respiratory depression. Of note, midazo-lam should not be prescribed for patients who have already been diagnosed with an existing allergy or with marked neuromuscular respiratory weakness including unstable myasthenia gravis, severe respira-tory depression, acute pulmonary insufficiency or sleep apnoea syndrome. If midazolam is prescribed with other central nervous system depressors, includ-ing tricyclic antidepressants, anticonvulsants or anti-psychotic drugs, it can result in enhanced sedation. Flumazenil is highly effective at reversing the effects of benzodiazepine-induced sedation and respiratory depression, and should be immediately available as an emergency drug in any area where midazolam is used.

Midazolam is administered prior to egg retrieval, usually as a standard dose of 2 mg IV.

4.4.2 Propofol

Although widely used in combination with other agents for oocyte retrieval [3], propofol is arguably

PRE-ASSESSMENT FORM

ACU Pre-Assessment

Name:	Consultant:
Address:	
Contact Number:	CHI:
	Gender:

Diabetes

Insulin ☐   drugs ☐   diet ☐   N/A ☐

☐ Obtain HbA1c   ☐ Diabetes + pregnancy leaflet given

Allergies   and   Reactions

Drugs	
Latex	
Other	

Medication (including inhalers/over the counter

Name (Generic)	Dose	Frequency	Comments (if medication held or stopped)

April 2014	Authorised		Page 1 of 4
Revision: 04			

Figure 4.1 A pre-operative assessment form developed for use in Ninewells Assisted Conception Unit (ACU).

PRE-ASSESSMENT FORM

Functional Activity Guide

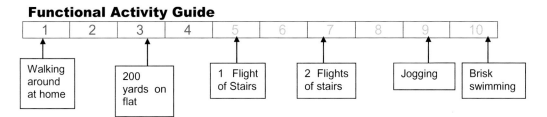

| 1 | 2 | 3 | 4 | 5 | 6 | 7 | 8 | 9 | 10 |

Walking around at home

200 yards on flat

1 Flight of Stairs

2 Flights of stairs

Jogging

Brisk swimming

Estimated METS score:
What prevents further activity?

Cardiovascular Assessment

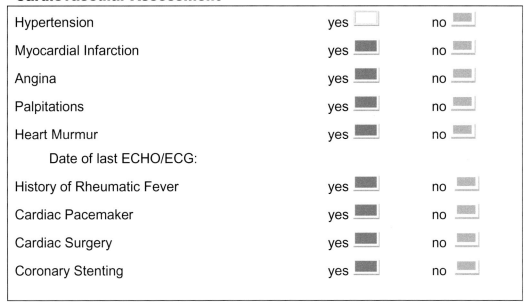

	yes	no
Hypertension	☐	▨
Myocardial Infarction	▨	▨
Angina	▨	▨
Palpitations	▨	▨
Heart Murmur	▨	▨
Date of last ECHO/ECG:		
History of Rheumatic Fever	▨	▨
Cardiac Pacemaker	▨	▨
Cardiac Surgery	▨	▨
Coronary Stenting	▨	▨

Figure 4.1 *(cont.)*

PRE-ASSESSMENT FORM

Respiratory Assessment

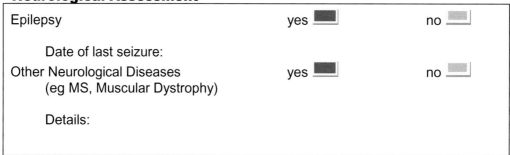

Smoker	yes ▇	no ☐
Asthma	yes ▇	no ▭
Hospital admission with asthma in past 3 years:	yes ▇	no ▭
Other Respiratory Disease	yes ▇	no ▭

Neurological Assessment

Epilepsy	yes ▇	no ▭
Date of last seizure:		
Other Neurological Diseases (eg MS, Muscular Dystrophy)	yes ▇	no ▭
Details:		

Other

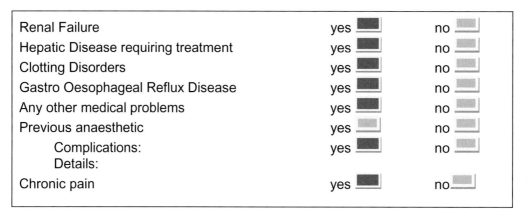

Renal Failure	yes ▇	no ▭
Hepatic Disease requiring treatment	yes ▇	no ▭
Clotting Disorders	yes ▇	no ▭
Gastro Oesophageal Reflux Disease	yes ▇	no ▭
Any other medical problems	yes ▇	no ▭
Previous anaesthetic	yes ▭	no ▭
Complications:	yes ▇	no ▭
Details:		
Chronic pain	yes ▇	no ▭

Figure 4.1 *(cont.)*

PRE-ASSESSMENT FORM

Observations

Pulse	**Regular**/Irregular (requires ECG) Sats %
BP	>140/90mmHg refer back to medical staff for advice
Weight:	kgs Height: BMI:

Signature: Date:

Notes

Any bold please refer to Nurse Sedationist for review

Figure 4.1 *(cont.)*

the single best sedation agent. Its exact mechanism of action is poorly understood, although it probably involves modulation of the inhibitory function of the neurotransmitter γ-aminobutyric acid (GABA). It provides rapid onset of sedation and anaesthesia, and has a short duration of action and efficient recovery with minimal drug accumulation. Due to its pharmacokinetic profile, a continuous infusion of propofol allows tight manipulation of sedation levels. It therefore delivers safe procedural sedation, short induction and recovery times, and high patient satisfaction [9].

In higher doses, propofol is a general anaesthetic agent, and its use can frequently precipitate cardiovascular and respiratory depression and rarely cardiac or respiratory arrest and death. For this reason, concern over the safety of propofol administration by health personnel without general anaesthetic training and airway management skills has arisen. Perhaps not unreasonably, the key controversy raised is that sedation is a continuum, margins of safety can easily be breached and training may be inadequate to rescue patients from deeper levels of sedation [10]. However, published literature supports the safety of conscious and deep sedation with propofol, including a retrospective case–control study, which included 6,840 patients undergoing 7,364 procedures [11].

Midazolam has a synergistic relationship with propofol. They are commonly co-administered to achieve conscious sedation. Their synergistic effect allows the use of smaller doses of both drugs, rather than a larger dose of one or the other. This is clearly beneficial, as it can help avoid side effects associated with higher doses of each individual drug [7].

Propofol 1% is administered using a target-controlled infusion pump, which is a syringe driver that can be programmed with a pre-designated treatment protocol. The Marsh model [12] is used for oocyte retrieval. In this model, compartmental volumes are proportional to weight, whereas rate constants for slow and fast redistribution are fixed. Once this protocol is selected, the weight and age of the patient is entered into the syringe driver. The infusion is commenced at 1 μg/ml and titrated to clinical effect. Titration to effect is critical to safely achieving sedation. However, the amount of propofol required to effectively sedate the patient for oocyte retrieval is influenced by both surgical and vaginal stimuli. As such, the infusion may need to be increased in response to stimulation but can also be reduced or discontinued as indicated [4].

4.4.3 Alfentanil

Alfentanil is a potent, short-acting opioid used primarily for its analgesic effects. Opioids act on the hypothalamus to decrease the body's response to stressful stimuli. The onset of action of alfentanil is rapid, with maximal analgesic and respiratory depressant effect occurring within 1–2 minutes. Due to its pharmacokinetic properties, it is an ideal painkiller for oocyte retrieval. It is quick acting and gives effective pain relief for acute episodes of pain, specifically insertion of the needle into the ovary, but does not have a long half-life, and thus does not cause long-lasting drowsiness and nausea compared with other opioids.

Co-administration with midazolam may also be of clinical benefit. Both drugs are metabolised by the same enzyme (cytochrome P450), and when used in combination, drug metabolism and clearance are more prolonged [13]. Patients therefore benefit from enhanced comfort and anxiolysis. With this delayed metabolism, however, the risks of respiratory depression are also increased. Opioids can also cause sedation and have a synergistic effect when given in combination with benzodiazepines. Naloxone can be used to treat symptoms of opioid overdose, including respiratory depression, and should be available in case of emergency.

In practice, 200 μg alfentanil is administered IV, and adequate time (1 minute) is allowed for it to be effective prior to commencing egg retrieval. Smaller bolus doses can be administered during the procedure for pain and discomfort.

4.4.4 Diclofenac

Diclofenac has anti-inflammatory, antipyretic and analgesic properties. It is effective in treating a variety of acute and chronic pain and inflammatory conditions and is the most frequently used non-steroidal anti-inflammatory drug (NSAID) globally [14]. As with all NSAIDs, diclofenac exerts its action by inhibition of cyclo-oxygenase and thus inhibition of prostaglandin synthesis. Research also suggests that diclofenac can inhibit the thromboxane prostanoid receptor, reduce arachidonic acid release and enhance arachidonic acid uptake, inhibit lipoxygenase enzymes, and activate the nitric oxide–cyclic guanosine monophosphate antinociceptive pathway [15]. Diclofenac 100 mg rectally is used most commonly following oocyte retrieval and offers up to 8 hours of pain relief post-administration.

Diclofenac inhibits platelet aggregation in vitro, but at therapeutic dosages, it has little effect on platelet aggregation, or prothrombin time. Nonetheless, administration of diclofenac is best avoided prior to oocyte retrieval in case of bleeding. Similarly, diclofenac is relatively contraindicated if heavy bleeding complicates oocyte retrieval.

4.5 Ovarian Hyperstimulation Syndrome

Although high doses of analgesia are not usually required for oocyte retrieval, patients with the potential for ovarian hyperstimulation syndrome (OHSS) due to high follicle numbers can experience increased abdominal discomfort during the procedure and therefore benefit from additional analgesia. In our experience, paracetamol prior to egg retrieval, either 1 g orally with the last drink before fasting, or 1 g IV, makes a difference not only to patient comfort during the procedure but also to recovery time and resulting discharge time.

The patient should be advised when their next dose of paracetamol can be taken prior to discharge. Alternatively, co-codamol may be advised for post-operative discomfort.

4.6 Monitoring and Oxygenation

Pulse oximetry, non-invasive blood pressure monitoring, electrocardiography and capnography are minimal requirements for safe monitoring for sedation [4] and should be continued until the patient is fully recovered. Patients receiving sedative medication must also have facial oxygen therapy administered [2].

Verbal monitoring is also mandatory during conscious sedation. The patient should maintain verbal communication throughout the procedure. However, because sedation is a continuum, it is not always possible to predict how an individual patient will respond. In the event that communication stops and the sedation level is deeper than intended, the propofol infusion should be reduced or discontinued and airway manoeuvres performed if indicated [2]. Emergency airway equipment and cardiovascular resuscitation equipment must always be available during sedation procedures, and staff should be trained in their use [16].

4.7 Post-sedation Care

Following oocyte retrieval, patient recovery should occur in a designated ward or room. This area must be staffed by those specifically trained in recovery and the patient monitored until fully recovered from sedation. Minimum observations should include heart rate, blood pressure, oxygen saturation and temperature. The conscious level of the patient must also be monitored and capnography used if the patient is deeply sedated.

During recovery, monitoring of pain scores is important, not only to ensure that the patient is comfortable following egg retrieval but also to detect any signs of post-operative complications, including bleeding. Adequate analgesia is also important because pain can delay discharge [17]. It is normal to experience minor abdominal cramps or pain following oocyte retrieval, and patients should be reassured that this usually settles quickly. Post-operative pain relief in the form of simple analgesia, for example paracetamol, is advised following discharge home. However, the patient should be given advice about worsening pain and advised to contact the fertility clinic should their pain increase or become unbearable.

Patients can be discharged as soon as an hour after completion of egg retrieval but should be accompanied home by an adult. This person is responsible for the patient's well-being, and should be advised to report any concerns following discharge. Post-sedation advice and post-operative analgesia should be given to the patient in front of the person taking responsibility for their care, as well as in writing [18]. It is important that the patient has a full understanding of this information and feels able to contact the department for advice or follow-up if required. The patient must be advised not to drive a vehicle or ride a bicycle or motorbike for 24 hours following sedation. They should also avoid operating machinery, or situations where impaired balance or co-ordination could be dangerous, and should avoid drinking alcohol as this could potentially cause serious side effects [2]. We also recommend that patients make arrangements for care of small children for 24 hours following sedation, and they should not sign any legally binding documents as their judgement may be impaired.

4.8 Nurse-Led Conscious Sedation

Nurse-led conscious sedation is provided routinely in many endoscopy units, and has been developed successfully for other services, including paediatrics [19]. However, this approach is uncommon in the fertility sector and, to our knowledge, there is no published clinical evidence regarding nurse-led conscious sedation for assisted conception procedures.

The importance of a multidisciplinary team in setting up and implementing a nurse-led conscious sedation service for oocyte retrieval is paramount. Effective planning, anaesthetic team involvement, training and support are key to the successful introduction of this approach into fertility services, with responsibility being delegated to nursing staff once competent. Pre-operative assessment tools, treatment protocols and patient information leaflets also need to be created.

Although the commonest sedative agents used in other areas are benzodiazepines, propofol is acknowledged to have the best outcomes for patient and physician satisfaction, as well as being more cost-effective [20]. While nurse administration of propofol is controversial, this can be achieved safely following appropriate training and with the use of capnography and target-controlled infusion pumps for administration. In our experience, the use of set protocols for nurse-led sedation and analgesia has ensured that all patients maintain verbal communication and therefore have a reduced risk of deep sedation, including during the recovery phase. Furthermore, clinical service evaluation has shown all-round benefits [21]. Trained nurse-led sedation is safe, effective and efficient, and nurses are motivated to undertake this extended role.

4.8.1 Sedation Protocols

Conscious sedation for oocyte retrieval is most commonly achieved using a combination of midazolam for anxiolysis, propofol for sedation and alfentanil for analgesia. However, concurrent administration of midazolam, propofol and alfentanil can potentially cause severe and life-threatening cardiovascular and respiratory depression. As part of the development of a nurse-led sedation service at Ninewells Assisted Conception Unit in Dundee (UK), sedation (Figure 4.2) and analgesia (Figure 4.3) protocols were created to allow safe drug administration by trained nurse sedationists. These include set limits for drugs.

Notably, the administration of one drug affects the timing and dose of administration of other drugs.

The skill of the nurse sedationist is to administer sedation and analgesia to allow oocyte retrieval to take place comfortably, but without the patient becoming oversedated and requiring airway or cardiovascular support. This requires constant vigilance and an understanding of oocyte retrieval, as well as knowledge of the relevant pharmacokinetics and pharmacodynamics. However, it is worth noting that adjuvant use of non-pharmacological management is also very important, and communication is an essential component of effective sedation. Speaking to the patient in a calm, effective and compassionate manner will provide reassurance and distraction, as well as complementing the effects of the sedation drugs [2]. Indeed, high patient satisfaction and good outcomes related to pain relief have been reported when the sedationist interacts with a patient in this manner.

4.8.2 Training

Anaesthetic training and assessment are required to provide appropriate skills for nurse sedationists. This includes practical skills training for IV access, vital sign monitoring and airway management, as well as knowledge-based learning in pharmacology, pre-operative assessment, airway management, recovery, management of emergencies and resuscitation. Advanced Life Support certification is essential prior to unsupervised practice, and, ideally, a non-medical prescriber qualification. Clinical teaching and assessment are an ongoing requirement for this post and should be supervised by the anaesthetic department.

The main priority of the nurse sedationist is the safety of the patient. Within NHS Tayside, there is an agreement that a named consultant anaesthetist is always available for support and advice to the nurse sedationist, and will provide rapid assistance, if required. Over time, the requirement of senior assistance has reduced, reflecting increasing experience and confidence of nurse sedation personnel working within rigorous policies and procedures.

4.8.3 Clinical Service Evaluation

Clinical service evaluation is an important tool for measuring current practice within a service, and can be used to drive improvement. It can also be used to

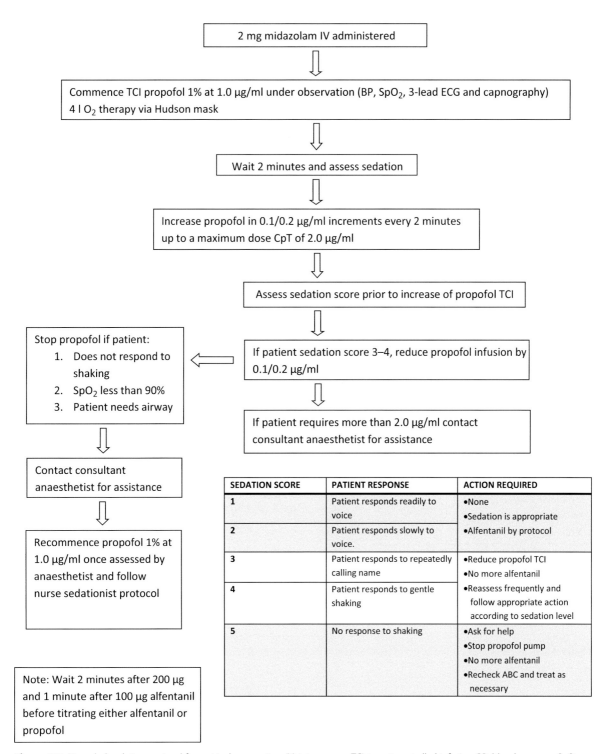

Figure 4.2 Nurse-led sedation protocol for assisted conception. IV, intravenous; TCI, target-controlled infusion; BP, blood pressure; SpO_2, oxygen saturation; ECG, electrocardiogram; Cpt, target plasma concentration;

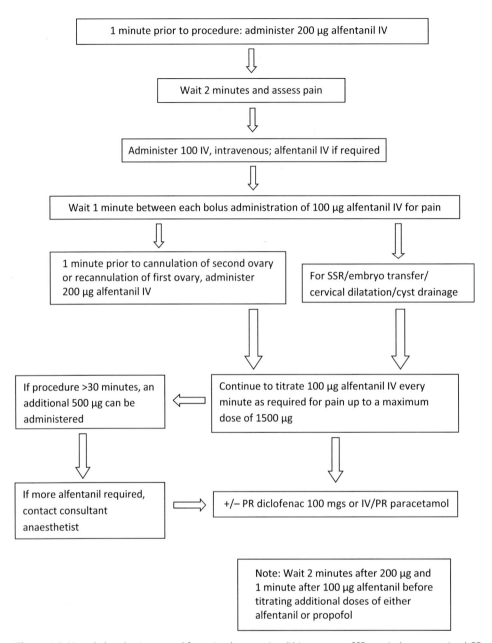

Figure 4.3 Nurse-led analgesia protocol for assisted conception. IV, intravenous; SSR, surgical sperm retrieval; PR, per rectum.

reflect upon an individual's practice, and can high-light areas for professional development. Quality evaluation is also an essential component of clinical governance and can be used to demonstrate that the nurse sedationist is maintaining standards and developing their practice.

Routinely collected data by the nurse-led sedation service should include recording the amount of drugs administered, time taken for the procedure and length of sedation, any adverse reactions including interventions required, never events and any occasions where assistance from a consultant anaesthetist is required. Clinical service evaluation demonstrates that nurse-administered sedation and analgesia protocols allow effective and pain-free oocyte retrieval [21]. Evidence also shows that 99% patients successfully undergo oocyte retrieval using these protocols, and that this is also an efficient approach, with a mean procedure length of 35 minutes from the start of sedation to return to recovery.

Our experience of nurse-led sedation has been very successful, due in part to its focus on the 'conscious' end of the sedation spectrum. Sedative medication and analgesia are administered, but equally, or perhaps more, important is patient rapport, dialogue and reassurance throughout the procedure. However, although our experience demonstrates the exceptional safety standards and successes of the nurse sedation role in NHS Tayside, it is important to point out that this approach would not be appropriate in a stand-alone unit without on-site consultant anaesthetist backup. Fertility clinics without appropriate immediate support should ensure that all anaesthesia and sedation are delivered by qualified and experienced anaesthetic personnel [16].

4.8.4 Challenges

As with any new service provision or development, initial assessment of nurse-led unsupervised practice

showed frequent minor late starts to egg collection. Although this did not impact on patient treatment outcomes, we recognised the need to adjust clinical practice to minimise this problem. By examining the patient pathway, process and timing of events occurring on the morning of oocyte retrieval, we made simple changes to streamline our working processes and reduce late starts. This positive impact on patient care also resulted in improved fertility teamwork.

4.9 Summary

Use of conscious sedation and analgesia is the commonest approach to provide pain relief during transvaginal oocyte retrieval. It is effective and has high levels of acceptability and patient satisfaction. Standards in safe sedation practice have been set out by the Royal College of Anaesthetists [4] and can be used to develop local guidelines appropriate to assisted conception [16]. Nurse-led sedation is appropriate and safe in the fertility sector, with certain caveats [21].

References

1. Kwan I, Wang R, Pearce E, Bhattacharya S. Pain relief for women undergoing oocyte retrieval for assisted reproduction. *Cochrane Database Syst Rev* 2018;**5**:CD004829. doi: 10.1002/14651858.CD004829.pub4

2. Academy of Medical Royal Colleges. *Safe Sedation for Healthcare Procedures: Standards and Guidance.* 2013. Available from: www.aomrc.org.uk/reports-guidance/safe-sedation-practice-1213/

3. Vlahos NF, Giannakikou I, Vlachos A, Vitoratos N. Analgesia and anesthesia for assisted reproductive technologies. *Int J Gynaecol Obstet* 2009;**105** (3):201–5. doi: 10.1016/j. ijgo.2009.01.017

4. Bailey CR, Ahuja M, Bartholomew K, et al. Guidelines for day-case surgery 2019: guidelines from the Association of

Anaesthetists and the British Association of Day Surgery. *Anaesthesia* 2019;**74**(6):778–92.

5. Zeinab H, Zohreh S, Gelehkolaee KS. Lifestyle and outcomes of assisted reproductive techniques: a narrative review. *Glob J Health Sci* 2015;**7**(4):11–22. doi: 10.5539/gjhs.v7n5p11

6. Pritchard MJ. Reducing anxiety in elective surgical patients. *Nurs Times* 2011;**107**(3):22–3.

7. Nuttall D, Rutt-Howard J. *The Textbook of Non-medical Prescribing*, 2nd ed. Hoboken, NJ: John Wiley & Sons, 2015.

8. Smith I, Kranke P, Murat I, et al. Perioperative fasting in adults and children: guidelines from the European Society of Anaesthesiology. *Eur J Anaesthesiol* 2011;**28**(8):556–69. doi: 10.1097/EJA.0b013e3283495ba1

9. Scarth E, Smith SP. *Drugs in Anaesthesia and Intensive Care,*

5th ed. Oxford: Oxford University Press, 2016.

10. Webb ST, Hunter DN. Is sedation by non-anaesthetists really safe? *Br J Anaesth* 2013;**111**(2):136–8. doi: 10.1093/bja/aet105

11. Jensen JT, Moller A, Hornslet P, Konge L, Vilmann P. Moderate and deep nurse-administered propofol sedation is safe. *Dan Med J* 2015;**62**(4):A5049.

12. Absalom AR, Mani V, de Smet T, Struys MM. Pharmacokinetic models for propofol – defining and illuminating the devil in the detail. *Br J Anaesth* 2009;**103** (1):26–37. doi: 10.1093/bja/aep143

13. Peck TE, Hill SA. *Pharmacology for Anaesthesia and Intensive Care*, 4th ed. Cambridge, UK: Cambridge University Press, 2014.

14. McGettigan P, Henry D. Use of non-steroidal anti-inflammatory drugs that elevate cardiovascular risk: an examination of sales and

essential medicines lists in low-, middle-, and high-income countries. *PLoS Med* 2013;**10**(2): e1001388. doi: 10.1371/journal. pmed.1001388

15. Gan TJ. Diclofenac: an update on its mechanism of action and safety profile. *Curr Med Res Opin* 2010;**26**(7):1715–31. doi: 10.1185/ 03007995.2010.486301

16. Acharya U, Elkington N, Manning L, Thorp-Jones D, Tavener G. Recommendations for good practice for sedation in assisted conception. *Hum Fertil (Camb)* 2020;**23**(3):150–8. doi: 10.1080/ 14647273.2019.1596245

17. Pavlin DJ, Chen C, Penaloza DA, Polissar NL, Buckley FP. Pain as a factor complicating recovery and discharge after ambulatory surgery. *Anesth Analg* 2002;**95** (3):627–34. doi: 10.1097/ 00000539-200209000-00025

18. Brattwall M, Stomberg MW, Jakobsson JG. [Ambulatory surgery in Sweden is structured and follows unified routines. A questionnaire on the practice of ambulatory surgery]. *Lakartidningen* 2012;**109** (41):1824–7.

19. Slynn C, Hulkes C. Developing a nurse-led child sedation service.

Nurs Child Young People 2012;**24** (6):20–2. doi: 10.7748/ ncyp2012.07.24.6.20.c9188

20. Tobias JD, Leder M. Procedural sedation: a review of sedative agents, monitoring, and management of complications. *Saudi J Anaesth* 2011;**5** (4):395–410. doi: 10.4103/1658- 354X.87270

21. Ulyatt J, Kay V. Fertility 2015: implementation of nurse sedation for assisted conception surgery. *Hum Fertil (Camb)* 2015;**18**:291–302. doi: 10.3109/ 14647273.2015.1060045.

Practical Clinical Aspects of Oocyte Retrieval

Peter I. Kerecsenyi and Raj Mathur

5.1 Introduction

Oocyte retrieval, also referred to as ovum pick up or egg collection, is a critical step in assisted conception treatment involving in vitro handling of oocytes. In this chapter, we consider how this step should be carried out, taking a clinical and practical approach.

5.2 Considerations before Oocyte Retrieval

5.2.1 Scheduling

Oocyte retrieval is usually timed for 34–38 hours after the trigger for final follicular maturation has been administered. In women with previous premature ovulation, the time interval may need to be shortened. When scheduling multiple patients, consideration must be given to the time it takes to complete each procedure. As the time of the trigger determines the time of oocyte retrieval, patients should be advised of their trigger times based on their position on the operating list. In most circumstances, triggers can be timed at 30–40-minute intervals, allowing the previous procedure to be completed. The number of patients who can have oocyte retrieval in one session depends on the capacity for the recovery and ward area. For oocyte retrieval under conscious sedation, recovery usually takes 2 hours; a five-bed ward would allow the list to proceed without interruption.

5.2.2 Preparation

Patients should be asked to arrive 60 minutes before the planned oocyte retrieval, allowing time for the necessary checks to be implemented.

It is good practice to confirm with the patient the time, type and dose of trigger administered, and whether any difficulties were experienced with it. Mistakes do happen: common ones are wrong timing of trigger injection, misunderstanding of the trigger

day or mis-administration of the injection. Hormone measurements to confirm that the trigger has been administered or has been effective are not part of routine care but may be useful in cases where there is a doubt. In the case of human chorionic gonadotropin (hCG) trigger, a simple urine pregnancy test is helpful: a negative result indicates lack of trigger. Serum β-hCG should be greater than 40 IU/l. In the case of an agonist trigger, the serum luteinising hormone level will be elevated [1].

After seeing the patient, the team involved in conducting the oocyte retrieval should participate in a safety brief. Problems such as mistakes with fasting, late arrival, a missing partner or interpreter and other factors may necessitate a change in the patient order. Anaesthetic concerns, such as severe chest infection, acid reflux or solid food intake within 6 hours may necessitate milder sedation or even require the procedure to be performed under local anaesthesia. A latex-free environment must be provided for patients with latex allergy. The equipment required should be specified, including whether a single- or double-channel needle is to be used. Any medical concerns and risk factors should be identified and discussed at the brief. It is good practice for a member of the laboratory staff to participate in the brief, and prior to starting the list, it should be confirmed that the laboratory is ready to receive eggs.

Before commencing the procedure, the surgeon and scrub staff should ensure that they have checked the equipment to be used and are happy with it. This includes the ultrasound machine, vacuum pump, heated stage and consumables.

5.2.3 Know Your Patient

The surgeon should ensure that the patient's medical notes are available and have been read. Records of previous oocyte retrieval may suggest difficult access to ovaries or a higher risk of bleeding. A history of previous oophorectomy should be noted, to avoid a fruitless search for an ovary that does not exist. Monitoring ultrasound scans performed during the cycle indicate the number and size of the follicles that need to be drained. Ultrasound can identify other potential issues such as ovarian cyst, endometrioma, hydrosalpinx or endometrial pathology. Difficulty in accessing the ovaries should be expected in the presence of large uterine fibroids and in cases where the ovary was difficult to visualise on transvaginal scanning. In most cases, a management plan should have been put in place prior to the day of oocyte retrieval.

Prior to proceeding with the procedure, the surgeon should ensure that the patient (and, if applicable, their partner) has given properly informed consent to all aspects of the treatment, including the oocyte retrieval procedure, gamete handling and legal parenthood. It is good practice to complete consent forms prior to the day of oocyte retrieval, and ideally before the treatment cycle starts. However, if this has not occurred, it is reasonable to obtain written informed consent on the day of oocyte retrieval, prior to the patient being sedated.

Any planned additional procedures should be discussed with the patient and consent obtained for these. Examples include a trial embryo transfer and drainage of a hydrosalpinx (see Chapter 6). Consider additional written consent especially for invasive procedures. Although at this point the patient should have a good understanding of the planned oocyte retrieval procedure (see Chapter 13), it is reassuring to hear the details from the surgeon; remind them that some abdominal discomfort and vaginal bleeding is quite common after the procedure.

5.2.4 The Patient's Perspective

Often, expectations and anxieties are focused on the oocyte retrieval as a climactic event in the treatment journey. A supportive, friendly atmosphere helps the patient to express any concerns. For many patients, this may be their first occasion of being in an operating theatre, while others may arrive with memories of previous painful procedures. Most of the anxieties are related to the fear of the unknown; a detailed explanation of the procedure during the preparation appointment, ward and theatre visit can help the patient to imagine the big day realistically (see Chapter 13).

Patients may feel uncomfortable or embarrassed by being exposed, while some patients feel unprotected without the presence of their partner. It is important to minimise the time and scale of exposure of the patient, and not have more staff than is necessary present in theatre. It is sensitive to ensure a female staff presence in the theatre.

The staff should take care to involve the partner in the conversations; they too may be worried about surgical complications and they have often less understanding of the procedure than the patient [2]. Building a trustful relationship with the anaesthetist is key to managing anxieties.

As for the whole fertility treatment process, honest and supportive management of expectations is critically important to achieving a satisfactory outcome. It is sensible to explain to patients prior to the procedure that the number of follicles does not translate directly into the number of eggs collected, and that finding empty follicles is also a possible outcome.

5.3 Considerations for the Theatre Routine

5.3.1 In Theatre

The identity of the patient should be checked. Identification of patients and traceability of their gametes is a crucial part of the IVF quality management system. A proper identification system should be in place using a unique identification code for each patient that refers to the patient's documentation and is used in the laboratory to label all devices containing biological material.

Patients should be asked directly to give their full name and date of birth before sedation starts. During this direct verification, the staff should check the corresponding unique identification code (patient ID against the ID code) and the correct labelling of the dishes (ID code against the label). This step should be witnessed by two members of staff, typically an embryologist and the surgeon. The use of an electronic identification system can minimise the risk of error in the laboratory, but the first step is direct verification. The same witnessed ID check should be performed before embryo transfer [3].

5.3.2 Sterility

Oocyte retrieval is a semi-sterile procedure. The preparation of the needle and the tubing and the fitting of the probe cover and needle guide should be done under aseptic conditions. The test tubes should be capped even when empty, and the rubber bung fitted to aspiration tubing must not contact any non-sterile surface in order to minimise contamination. The plastic needle cover should be removed only as a very last step before oocyte retrieval starts. Both the surgeon and scrub assistant should wear sterile gloves and a protective apron.

5.3.3 Patient Positioning

The patient should be in lithotomy position. The hips should be positioned at the edge of the operating table so that the scan probe can be moved freely, allowing access even if the ovaries are positioned high or very anteriorly. The position may need to be adapted to patient mobility. The lower limbs should be covered by sterile drapes both to reduce risk of contamination and to respect the patient's dignity.

5.3.4 Vaginal Preparation

During oocyte retrieval, the needle is inserted through the vaginal wall with the theoretical risk of bacterial transmission into the pelvis. Fortunately, infection complications such as pelvic abscess are rare, irrespective of whether prophylactic antibiotics or vaginal disinfection are used.

There is insufficient evidence on which to base recommendations regarding vaginal disinfection prior to needle insertion. Normal saline is commonly used to cleanse the vagina. Patients with pelvic endometriosis, especially with endometrioma, are at increased risk of developing severe pelvic inflammatory disease, including pelvic abscess after oocyte retrieval [4]. In these cases, the use of povidone iodine followed by a saline wash may be considered.

A prospective study showed that povidone iodine was associated with a significantly lower clinical pregnancy rate [5]. As a result, it is not recommended for routine use. Later studies suggested that subsequent saline douching can prevent such a harmful effect, but these studies did not prove that routine povidone iodine use could prevent formation of pelvic abscess [6–8].

5.3.5 Antibiotic Prophylaxis

The incidence of significant pelvic infection following oocyte retrieval is in the range of 0.4–1.3%. There is insufficient evidence to make recommendations concerning the use of antibiotic prophylaxis in low-risk patients, and practice varies among different clinics.

Studies have identified groups of women who are at an increased risk of pelvic infection, including those with a history of pelvic inflammatory disease, hydrosalpinx and endometriosis. While there is no comparative evidence in these groups, it is reasonable to take a precautionary approach and provide prophylactic antibiotics.

The principles to follow include choice of appropriate agent and administration prior to the start of the procedure, to achieve tissue levels at the time of needle passage through the vagina and into the ovaries. In order to obtain adequate tissue levels, oral antibiotics need to be started several hours prior to the procedure, while intravenous antibiotics may be administered in theatre at the start of sedation.

Cases of severe pelvic infection have been reported in high-risk women despite the use of prophylactic antibiotics. Hence, patients must be counselled about the symptoms of pelvic infection and asked to report urgently if they develop fever, malaise, abdominal pain or vaginal discharge, for a full clinical evaluation.

5.4 Equipment Required for Oocyte Retrieval

5.4.1 Ultrasound Scan Machine

Oocyte retrieval is routinely guided by a conventional two-dimensional transvaginal ultrasound probe. A three-dimensional ultrasound scan has no real additional value and is time consuming. Although rarely required, an abdominal transducer should also be at hand in case of unusual anatomy or if the ovaries cannot be seen on transvaginal scanning. The scan machine should be equipped with the option to display the needle guideline on the screen and possess the ability to print and save images. This should be done before the procedure starts.

The machine should be tested and set up before the first case of the day. The centre should have an emergency plan in case of machine or transducer fault. (Remember that the transducer is manufacturer specific and so is the needle guide; the backup scan/transducer may need a different needle guide!)

The vaginal ultrasound probe is covered by a specific sterile probe cover, which is long enough to cover the entire probe. A small amount of ultrasound gel is applied to the tip of the transducer under but not on the outside of the probe cover. Take care not to trap air bubbles under the probe cover as these may impair the image. Do not use lubricant as it may be toxic to the oocytes.

Single-use, disposable needle guides are available for transducers of most major manufacturers. Reusable guides need meticulous brush cleaning and sterilisation in order to avoid contamination or blockage.

Care should be taken to fit the needle guide properly onto the transducer. Improper fitting will guide the needle askew, so it will not follow the guideline on the screen, leading to the risk of inadvertent visceral or vascular injury.

5.4.2 Temperature Control

Oocytes are extremely sensitive to pH changes and transient cooling in vitro. Even modest fluctuations in temperature can cause disruption of the meiotic spindle with possible chromosome dispersal and also abnormal oocyte activation [9].

The test tubes used to collect follicular fluid should therefore be kept at or close to 37°C. One test tube full of flushing medium per patient should be pre-warmed in the laboratory and its temperature should be kept at 37°C in the test-tube heater at all times.

It is practical to choose a test-tube heater with a transparent front panel, which enables continuous observation of the fluid level. A removable panel makes cleaning simple. Continuous temperature measurement is useful – this can be achieved using a simple immersible temperature sensor in a test tube, filled with water, connected to a digital display that is in sight at all times.

Test tubes containing follicular fluid should be transported to the laboratory in the shortest possible time and with the least temperature disruption. A heated test-tube block is useful for this purpose. In the laboratory, a temperature-controlled workstation where the fluid is examined in dishes on a heated plate minimises any temperature fluctuations.

5.4.3 Aspiration Needles

Aspiration needles are available in different diameters, ranging from 15 to 20 gauge. A needle with a larger diameter is more rigid (will not bend), easier to follow on the screen and allows greater flow rate

(shorter operating time), while a smaller diameter needle causes less discomfort, so could be a choice for cases with minimal anaesthesia. The needle length varies between 300 and 350 mm, and the length of the attached aspiration tubing between 40 and 100 cm. Shorter tubing reduces temperature fluctuation and the risk of cumulus–oocyte complex (COC) damage, while a longer tubing allows much more comfortable work with easy manoeuvrability of the needle.

Both the needle length and internal diameter influence the required aspiration pressure (vacuum). For a long needle with small diameter, a higher aspiration pressure is required to achieve a good flow rate. The higher pressure and increased velocity may damage the oocyte. The manufacturer's instructions about the suction pressure settings should be adhered to.

Aspiration needles with an echogenic tip are preferred, as this enhances visualisation on the ultrasound screen and helps depth control.

Should we use single- or double-lumen aspiration needles? During oocyte retrieval using a single-lumen needle, fluid is removed from the follicles by aspiration in one direction. Oocytes are recovered from around 80% of follicles aspirated, although this rate varies from patient to patient. With a double-lumen needle, follicular flushing can be carried out. These needles allow injection of flushing medium through a second lumen into the follicle. This may add to the operative time, and the wider diameter of a double-lumen needle may increase patient discomfort.

5.4.4 To Flush or Not To Flush?

Although the use of follicular flushing is quite widespread, the available evidence does not support its routine use. A Cochrane review found that, in normal responders, follicular flushing was not associated with improvements in live birth rate, clinical pregnancy rate, oocyte yield, total number of embryos or the number of embryos cryopreserved [10].

Similar conclusions were drawn for poor responders where five or fewer follicles were seen on the day of hCG trigger [11]. The mean number of COC or the number of mature oocytes did not increase with flushing. The proportion of randomised patients having at least one COC retrieved was no different between groups. No difference was observed between groups for mean number of embryos, the proportion of randomised patients achieving embryo transfer, clinical pregnancy and live birth rates. Based on these findings, National Institute for Health and Care Excellence (NICE) guidelines do not recommend the use of follicular flushing when at least three follicles have developed before oocyte retrieval [12].

In a small group of patients – extreme poor responders, natural cycle or modified natural cycle patients where only between one and three follicles are present – flushing may be justified. The retrieval of at least one oocyte may determine whether embryo transfer occurs at all. One study observed that cumulative oocyte recovery rate was significantly increased after up to four flushes, and oocytes did not differ regarding maturity, fertilisation rate or embryo quality [13].

5.4.5 Flushing the Tubing System

Once the tubing system is connected to the first test tube and to the pump, and you are ready to start the actual oocyte retrieval, flush through the tubing with flushing medium. This step is important for three reasons: (1) it further reduces the risk of temperature fluctuation while the oocytes are travelling; (2) it reduces the risk of turbulent flow, which could damage the COC; and (3) it confirms that your system is working.

It requires around 2–3 ml of flushing medium to fill up the system. The content of the first tube will be largely clear medium before the follicular fluid starts to come through. Similarly, at the end of oocyte retrieval, proper flushing will empty the rest of the follicular fluid from the tubing system.

5.5 The Technique of Oocyte Retrieval

5.5.1 Description of the Procedure

Before starting to scan for oocyte retrieval, the checklist shown in Table 5.1 should be followed.

Insert the scan probe carefully, take care that the edge of the probe cover does not hit the urinary meatus.

Start with an orientation scan of the uterus, adnexa, ovaries and urinary bladder. Record any free fluid, unusual ovarian findings or fluid in the uterine cavity.

Set the zoom so that the full depth of the ovary can be seen. Set the gain to optimise picture quality.

Check the prospective track of the aspiration needle journey: is there anything in its route to the

Table 5.1. Checklist before starting to scan for oocyte retrieval

The tubing system is set up and connected.

Tube heater is providing 37°C heat and pre-warmed flushing medium is prepared.

A sufficient number of test tubes are prepared.

The vacuum pump is tested.

The scan machine is set with the needle guideline on screen, and the patient selected if required.

The vagina is cleansed and the patient is covered.

The scan probe is prepared with ultrasound gel, and probe cover and needle guide attached.

Anaesthesia is applied as planned.

Urinary catheter with kidney dish/sick bowl, packs of sterile gauze, emergency suture pack.

ovary? Structures include the venous plexus, broad ligament, bladder, bowel (particularly in cases of endometriosis) and even the iliac artery. A cystic structure (e.g. follicle or ovarian cyst) may be distinguished from a tubular structure (e.g. vessel or hydrosalpinx) by rotating the scan probe through 90°. Empty the bladder if necessary, if it is intervening between the vaginal fornix and the ovary.

It makes sense to begin the oocyte retrieval on the side with the easier access. Scan through the whole ovary to find the area for the most direct access and least risk of injury. Colour Doppler may be helpful to avoid vessels. Press the probe firmly against the fornix and keep it tight through the whole procedure. This will help stabilise the ovaries and prevent structures from moving into the path of the needle.

Next, the needle is inserted through the needle guide and through the vaginal wall. The probe should always be inserted fully first, and the needle second. Inserting the scan probe with the needle already in the needle guide channel creates the risk of an anterior vaginal wall tear with potentially severe bleeding. Ensure that the needle follows the guideline on the ultrasound screen.

Start the aspiration pump and lead the needle through into the middle of a follicle. Once the follicle has collapsed, gently rotate the needle to allow all the fluid to empty. Keep the pump running while the needle is removed from the follicle to prevent reverse flow and potential loss of follicular fluid. (Some pumps are equipped with a valve control to avoid reverse flow.) You can operate the pump continuously while the needle is in the ovary. Make sure, however, that the pump is off before the needle tip leaves the ovary to avoid air being sucked in, as frothing may cause turbulence with a risk of damaging the COC.

Keep checking both the scan picture and test tube as the follicle is aspirated. Try to empty the contents of one follicle into one test tube: interrupting the vacuum may cause leakage of the follicular fluid at the needle entry. The assistant, who is handling the test tubes, must remain vigilant at all times to prevent overflow with the potential loss of follicular fluid and eggs.

Make sure you move the needle under full visual control. In order to reach all the follicles, withdraw the needle inside the ovarian tissue before you change the angle of the scan probe. Usually, all follicles can be reached from one or two vaginal wall punctures, unless the ovaries are very large or awkwardly located.

An effort should be made to empty all accessible follicles. Follicles sized over 13 mm will most probably provide an oocyte, but more than 50% of the 8–13 mm-sized follicles (0.3–0.9 ml) will be also active, leading to blastocysts and pregnancies in a comparable rate to larger follicles [14]. Once all the follicles have been emptied, remove the needle and apply a final flush.

At the end of the procedure, a further scan survey should be carried out. The surgeon should compare the amount and echodensity of free fluid with that seen at the start and look for active bleeding.

Both adnexa should be scanned to exclude hydrosalpinx: even if it was not seen before, the enlarged ovaries may have obstructed the fimbrial end causing fluid to accumulate. The finding of a hydrosalpinx may indicate the need for elective cryopreservation of all embryos and investigation (see Chapter 6).

The scan should also measure endometrial thickness and morphology, and any irregularities or fluid in the cavity. Endometrial fluid in a fresh cycle is most often transient and disappears by the time of embryo transfer and will not affect pregnancy rates. In the case of persistent fluid, 'freeze all' may be advised, although several pregnancies have been reported after aspiration of fluid immediately before embryo transfer [15].

Finally, the vagina is cleaned using a sponge on a sponge-holder and a sanitary pad applied.

5.5.2 Oocyte Retrieval for In Vitro Maturation

For in vitro maturation, immature oocytes are collected from antral follicles. These follicles are typically sized 2–8 mm. The general consensus is to deliver the trigger when three follicles reach a size of greater than 6 mm but no follicle is larger than 13 mm. Oocyte retrieval is timed at 36–38 hours after trigger. Very small follicle volumes and more common bleeding make oocyte retrieval challenging. A double-channel aspiration needle is routinely used [16].

5.5.3 Technique of Follicular Flushing

In preparation, a non-toxic 20 ml syringe should be filled with pre-warmed flushing medium and the tubing system should first be flushed through. In this way, injecting air into the follicle can be avoided, which would cause irregular pressure levels. Keeping the syringe in the palm can reduce temperature drop. It requires some practice to handle the scan probe, needle and syringe at the same time, but this allows synchronised work between the syringe and the pump. Alternatively, the assistant can handle the syringe.

Once the follicular fluid has been aspirated, the follicle collapses. At this point, the pump is stopped and the needle kept steady *in situ*. The flushing medium is injected gradually and the follicle is seen to re-expand. Care should be taken not to expand the follicle beyond its original size. The pump is then restarted to empty the follicle again. These steps are repeated two to three times, unless an oocyte is obtained prior to that. It is useful to bear in mind the latency due to 2–3 ml of dead space in the needle and the tubing system.

5.6 Common Difficulties during Oocyte Retrieval

5.6.1 Endometrioma and Other Cysts

Endometriomas should not be punctured unless this is essential to access follicles. Fluid from endometriomas contains high levels of cell damage-mediating factors such as proteolytic enzymes, inflammatory mediators and reactive oxygen species, which are toxic to the oocytes and to the ovarian tissue. The thick fluid may block the needle. If the fluid leaks from the cyst, it may cause an inflammatory reaction, often followed by extensive adhesion formation. Pelvic abscess has been reported as complication.

If an endometrioma is punctured accidentally, it is preferable to use a new needle and tubing set to finish oocyte retrieval, or at least to apply thorough flushing.

Thin-walled simple cysts are often difficult to differentiate from follicles during oocyte retrieval. It is reasonable to drain such cysts. Obviously, large (>50 mm) or suspicious cysts must be investigated prior to stimulation or – if identified during stimulation – they should be left undrained during oocyte retrieval for appropriate investigation.

5.6.2 Difficulty in Accessing the Ovaries

Sometimes, it is difficult to reach the ovary. Some measures that may be useful in this situation are as follows: manipulating the transducer head into the vaginal fornix, a change in patient position (reverse Trendelenburg or lateral tilt), and external manual pressure through the abdominal wall to move the ovary closer to the vagina or to keep it fixed if it is too mobile.

The obstacle is often the uterus: due to pelvic adhesions or to an enlarged, distorted uterus, there may be no other way to reach the ovary than through the myometrium. In a report, transmyometrial oocyte retrieval was found as the only option in 1.7% of 5,115 cases [17]. A standard oocyte retrieval needle was passed through the myometrium and the fundal endometrium was carefully avoided. No bleeding complications were reported from any of the 85 cases and ongoing pregnancy rate was not affected.

When transmyometrial oocyte retrieval seems the only available option, careful assessment is necessary. The surgeon should try to avoid the arcuate arteries as well as the uterine cavity. The main limitation of the technique is that the needle mobility is massively reduced owing to the density of the myometrium. It is sensible to avoid multiple punctures of the uterus.

If the ovaries cannot be accessed transvaginally, a transabdominal ultrasound-guided approach is an option but carries a risk of bowel and vascular injury. In our practice, we prefer a laparoscopic approach in such cases, allowing direct visualisation of the ovaries. This is particularly useful in cases of pelvic adhesions and large fibroids, where the ovaries are displaced out of the pelvis and have limited mobility, as well as in cases of uterovaginal agenesis. In most units, laparoscopic oocyte retrieval is not possible as a 'rescue'

measure, which highlights the importance of accurate ultrasound assessment of ovarian access during monitoring.

When performing laparoscopic oocyte retrieval, the suction needle may be introduced directly through the abdominal wall under vision, or through a 5 mm port (suprapubic or lateral). Direct insertion may cause the needle to bend and become unusable, particularly in an obese patient. Insertion through a port causes some inevitable loss of pneumoperitoneum. In contrast to ultrasound-guided aspiration, laparoscopic aspiration of ovarian follicles requires the surgeon to estimate proprioceptively the depth of penetration of the needle to ensure all follicles are drained, without traversing the ovary. In our practice, we aspirate any pelvic free fluid at the end of the procedure, in case oocytes have been shed from the ovary.

It is reported that in cases of unilateral oocyte retrieval where the second ovary was not accessible, the chance of achieving at least one good-quality blastocyst, clinical pregnancy rate and live birth rate were not affected, provided at least five oocytes were collected [18]. This observation suggests that once a reasonable number of eggs have been collected from the accessible ovary, patient safety should be preferred over oocyte number. Undue risks should not be taken in such circumstances.

5.6.3 Bleeding during Oocyte Retrieval

Follicles have rich vascularity and small amount of bleeding during oocyte retrieval is usually unavoidable (see Chapter 7). The blood can be seen to refill the follicle, giving a more echodense content compared with follicular fluid. This bleeding is almost always self-limiting and does not cause concern.

Thicker branches of the ovarian artery are usually in the central, medulla part of the ovary but there is no reliable technique available to avoid vessels [19]. The uterine artery forms a rich anastomosis with the vaginal and the ovarian artery. A dilated venous plexus is often seen, especially in parous patients. Injury of these vessels will cause intraperitoneal or, rarely, subperitoneal bleeding. Using colour Doppler may help to identify the source of arterial bleeding. The bleeding will stop usually within a few minutes.

The external iliac vein or artery is often visible behind or around the ovary, sometimes running quite medially. Obviously, these must be avoided. Typically, there is a risk of large-vessel injury when the ovary is mobile and the surgeon tries to enter a distal follicle by a sudden, rapid needle movement, without precise depth control.

The cervical branches of the uterine artery are close to the fornix: these are usually the source of vaginal bleeding. It sometimes can be quite heavy; applying firm pressure of a sponge with a sponge holder for 3–5 minutes is usually sufficient to stop it. On rare occasions, a suture may be necessary; an emergency suture pack containing a small curved needle, absorbable suture, needle holder and long scissors should be available in theatre.

5.7 After the Procedure

The post-procedure monitoring and the discharge process are detailed in Chapter 8 and management of complications in Chapter 7.

After oocyte retrieval, the risk of ovarian hyperstimulation syndrome should be reassessed, and relevant prophylactic measures should be advised. These may include elective cryopreservation of all embryos and continued use of a gonadotropin-releasing hormone antagonist.

In cases where no oocyte was collected in poor responders, rescue intrauterine insemination can be considered, assuming there is suitable sperm quality and at least one patent Fallopian tube. The insemination should be delivered within a few hours of oocyte retrieval. The risk of multiple pregnancy should be carefully considered. As it might be problematic to gain valid consent after sedation, it is good practice to discuss with such patient the option of rescue insemination before oocyte retrieval. Additional consent may be required from the partner for different use of sperm.

References

1. Matorras R, Meabe A, Mendoza R, et al. Human chorionic gonadotropin (hCG) plasma levels at oocyte retrieval and IVF outcomes. *J Assist Reprod Genet* 2012;**29**: 1067–71. doi: 10.1007/s10815-012-9826-7

2. Schaller MA, Griesinger G, Banz-Jansen C. Women show a higher level of anxiety during IVF treatment than men and hold different concerns: a cohort study. *Arch Gynecol Obstet* 2016;**293** (5):1137–45. doi: 10.1007/s00404-016-4033-x

3. European Society of Human Reproduction and Embryology (ESHRE). *The Revised Guidelines for Good Practice in IVF Laboratories (2015)*. Strombeek-Bever, Belgium: ESHRE, 2015. Available from: www.eshre.eu/Guidelines-and-Legal/Guidelines/Revised-guidelines-for-good-practice-in-IVF-laboratories-(2015).aspx

4. Elizur SE, Lebovitz O, Weintraub AY, et al. Pelvic inflammatory disease in women with endometriosis is more severe than in those without. *Aust N Z J Obstet Gynaecol* 2014;**54**(2):162–5. doi: 10.1111/ajo.12189

5. van Os HC, Roozenburg BJ, Janssen-Caspers HA, et al. Vaginal disinfection with povidone iodine and the outcome of in-vitro fertilization. *Hum Reprod* 1992;7 (3):349–50. doi: 10.1093/oxfordjournals.humrep.a137647

6. Tsai YC, Lin MY, Chen SH, et al. Vaginal disinfection with povidone iodine immediately before oocyte retrieval is effective in preventing pelvic abscess formation without compromising the outcome of IVF-ET. *J Assist Reprod Genet* 2005;**22**(4):173–5. doi: 10.1007/s10815-005-4915-5

7. Hannoun A, Awwad J, Zreik T, Ghaziri G, Abu-Musa A. Effect of betadine vaginal preparation during oocyte aspiration in in vitro fertilization cycles on pregnancy outcome. *Gynecol Obstet Invest* 2008;**66**(4):274–8. doi: 10.1159/000156378

8. Funabiki M, Taguchi S, Hayashi T, et al. Vaginal preparation with povidone iodine disinfection and saline douching as a safe and effective method in prevention of oocyte pickup-associated pelvic inflammation without spoiling the reproductive outcome: evidence from a large cohort study. *Clin Exp Obstet Gynecol* 2014;**41** (6):689–90.

9. Almeida PA, Bolton VN. The effect of temperature fluctuations on the cytoskeletal organisation and chromosomal constitution of the human oocyte. *Zygote* 1995;**3** (4):357–65. doi: 10.1017/s0967199400002793

10. Georgiou EX, Melo P, Brown J, Granne IE. Follicular flushing during oocyte retrieval in assisted reproductive techniques. *Cochrane Database Syst Rev* 2018;**4**:CD004634. doi: 10.1002/14651858.CD004634.pub3

11. Neumann K, Griesinger G. Follicular flushing in patients with poor ovarian response: a systematic review and meta-analysis. *Reprod Biomed Online* 2018;**36**(4):408–15. doi: 10.1016/j.rbmo.2017.12.014

12. National Institute for Health and Care Excellence (NICE). *Fertility Problems: Assessment and Treatment. Clinical Guideline CG156*. London: NICE, 2013. Available from: www.nice.org.uk/guidance/cg156

13. Xiao Y, Wang Y, Wang M, Liu K. Follicular flushing increases the number of oocytes retrieved in poor ovarian responders undergoing in vitro fertilization: a retrospective cohort study. *BMC Women's Health* 2018;**18** (1):186. doi: 10.1186/s12905-018-0681-2

14. Wirleitner B, Okhowat J, Vištejnová L, et al. Relationship between follicular volume and oocyte competence, blastocyst development and live-birth rate: optimal follicle size for oocyte retrieval. *Ultrasound Obstet Gynecol* 2018;**51**(1):118–25. doi: 10.1002/uog.18955

15. Gupta N, Bhandari S, Agrawal P, Ganguly I, Singh A. Effect of endometrial cavity fluid on pregnancy rate of fresh versus frozen in vitro fertilization cycle. *J Hum Reprod Sci* 2017;**10** (4):288–92. doi: 10.4103/0974-1208.223282

16. Rose BI. Approaches to oocyte retrieval for advanced reproductive technology cycles planning to utilize in vitro maturation: a review of the many choices to be made. *J Assist Reprod Genet* 2014;**31**(11):1409–19. doi: 10.1007/s10815-014-0334-9

17. Davis LB, Ginsburg ES. Transmyometrial oocyte retrieval and pregnancy rates. *Fertil Steril* 2004;**81**(2):320–2. doi: 10.1016/j. fertnstert.2003.06.019

18. Olgan S, Mumusoglu S, Bozdag G. Does unilateral oocyte retrieval due to transvaginally inaccessible ovaries, contrary to common beliefs, affect IVF/ICSI treatment outcomes that much? *Biomed Res Int* 2016;**2016**:3687483. doi: 10.1155/2016/3687483

19. Rísquez F, Confino E. Can Doppler ultrasound-guided oocyte retrieval improve IVF safety? *Reprod Biomed Online* 2010;**21**:444–5. doi: 10.1016/j. rbmo.2010.04.035

Challenges during Oocyte Retrieval

Stephen Davies and Mostafa Metwally

6.1 Difficult Ovarian Access

Since its introduction in the 1980s, transvaginal ultrasound-guided oocyte retrieval (TVOR) has become the most widely accepted method worldwide of accessing the ovaries and retrieving oocytes for use in in vitro fertilisation (IVF). This technique allows safe and relatively easy access to the ovaries in the vast majority of women undergoing treatment. However, in 1–2% of women, access via this route proves technically challenging and may or not be achieved using a variety of manoeuvres [1].

In most cases, this impaired accessibility should be established well in advance of the procedure and treatment plans adjusted to compensate for these problems. There will still be occasions, however, when difficult access is encountered when doing a TVOR procedure and this had not been anticipated.

Most cases of difficult access will relate to the formation of previous adhesions, particularly from pelvic inflammatory disease or endometriosis. Larger uterine fibroids can also commonly affect access to the ovaries. Previous pelvic or abdominal surgery, especially if related to a perforated viscus or inflammatory bowel disease, is also likely to affect the mobility and position of the ovaries and therefore their suitability for TVOR.

Other cases, albeit rare, will relate to congenital abnormalities, which may make transvaginal access impossible, and other options for access will need to be considered from the outset of treatment.

6.1.1 Management

6.1.1.1 Emptying the Bladder

It is important to ensure that the bladder is empty prior to commencing the procedure. The relative positions of the uterus and ovaries can be significantly altered by the amount of urine in the bladder, and it is standard practice to ask patients to empty their bladder immediately prior to TVOR. However, some patients have poor bladder sensation, and it will often be seen on the scan that there is a considerable residual volume within the bladder; in addition, during any procedure, the rate of bladder filling can be very variable. As such, use of a disposable catheter to fully empty the bladder can significantly improve access to the ovaries.

6.1.1.2 Position of the Probe

Altering the position of the transvaginal probe can improve accessibility, and this is often augmented by the use of simultaneous abdominal pressure from an assistant. The ovary may be accessed using a different trajectory and, provided the user is confident of avoiding damage to any adjacent structures, especially the bowel and blood vessels, this can be safely achieved. Use of colour Doppler ultrasound can help avoid vascular trauma. Occasionally, changing the patient's position can help, including the use of a table tilt to assist access.

6.1.1.3 Use of a Tenaculum

Applying downward traction on the cervix with a tenaculum can in a limited number of cases improve access to the ovaries.

6.1.1.4 Transmyometrial Access of the Ovaries

In some cases, the ovary is fixed posteriorly to the uterus and there is little, if any, movement with any of the manoeuvres listed above. The only way to rescue the cycle in terms of oocyte retrieval from that ovary is to consider whether to access the ovary via a transmyometrial approach, and this has been done successfully with resulting pregnancies [2]. Avoiding the fundal region is advised, and there should also be an awareness of the increased likelihood of needle blockage with thick tissue. Use of positive pressure during needle transit can be helpful.

6.1.1.5 Transabdominal Ultrasound-Guided or Laparoscopic Oocyte Retrieval

In rare cases, the operator will need to consider a transabdominal ultrasound-guided or laparoscopic oocyte retrieval.

Transabdominal Ultrasound-Guided Oocyte Retrieval

Before the introduction of TVOR, transabdominal ultrasound-guided oocyte retrieval was a commonly practised technique. This technique can often be performed immediately when transvaginal ultrasound is found to be non-feasible (although accessibility to the ovaries should always be assessed during cycle monitoring, hence allowing time to plan for alternative approaches if needed). After the use of suitable anaesthesia (local infiltration, spinal or general anaesthetic) and cleaning of the abdominal wall, the abdominal wall is penetrated with the oocyte needle in the usual way, but, given the limited elasticity of the abdominal wall, several punctures are often needed [3]. Apart from being associated with a slightly lower number of retrieved oocytes, transabdominal oocyte retrieval has been found to be a safe and effective technique [3].)

Laparoscopic Oocyte Retrieval

In contrast to transabdominal ultrasound-guided oocyte retrieval, a laparoscopic approach requires prior planning. Flexible protocols for ovarian stimulation such as the long agonist protocol are often necessary to allow flexibility with surgical planning (e.g. booking theatre space and date). The laparoscopic approach is particularly indicated in women with significant congenital anomalies such as Müllerian agenesis or where the ovary is fixed in a high position and cannot be accessed vaginally, despite all the techniques previously mentioned. Although transabdominal ultrasound-guided oocyte retrieval is also possible in such cases, this is often difficult, especially in cases where the anatomy is significantly distorted and the ovaries are difficult to safely identify or access due to overlying bowel. In women with Müllerian agenesis in particular, the ovaries are often located in a position above the pelvic brim with overlying loops of bowel and in close proximity to the major pelvic vessels at the pelvic brim. In such cases, identification and access of the ovaries is often safer laparoscopically.

Laparoscopic oocyte egg collection is a relatively straightforward procedure for the average laparoscopic surgeon, as long as the operator is aware of what to expect during the procedure. Accessing the ovaries is done using the standard needles placed down the secondary laparoscopic ports. It is first important to identify the exact position of the ovaries, as this will dictate the site of insertion of the secondary ports; for example, ovaries located in a high position above the pelvic brim in women with Müllerian agenesis may require higher insertion of the lateral ports rather than the standard position in the iliac fossae. After identification of the ovaries, the operator inserts the needle down the ports and penetrates the follicles in the usual way. Alternatively, the operator might find it easier to access both ovaries from a single midline port, such as a suprapubic port. Although the needle may also be placed directly through the skin, due to the thickness of the abdominal wall, the needle can easily become obstructed by tissue from the anterior abdominal wall.

When performing the procedure for the first time, the operator may be surprised by how vascular the stimulated ovary appears and by how common it is to see the follicles fill with blood after aspiration. This is what normally happens at any transvaginal oocyte retrieval, but seeing the effects on an ultrasound screen is different from the real picture seen at laparoscopy. The operator should therefore avoid the temptation to apply diathermy or suture any bleeding points, as this may lead to disastrous consequences given the friability and vascularity of the ovary. For the same reason, ovarian manipulations with laparoscopic instruments should be kept to a minimum and performed very gently.

6.2 Bleeding Complications

Significant bleeding at the time of TVOR is a very rare occurrence. Studies have shown an incidence of between 2.8 and 8% [4], but in the vast majority of these cases, this is minor bleeding that does not need any active intervention or resuscitation. Life-threatening bleeding probably occurs in fewer than 1 in 1,000 cases. Obviously, the existence of underlying bleeding disorders or medication that affects haemostasis will significantly alter the risk of this complication. Prevention is absolutely the key to management of this condition, as in the vast majority of cases it is entirely avoidable.

Technique and operator experience is vital to minimise the risk of significant bleeding. Careful scanning in both axes throughout the pelvis is crucial to assess whether the aspiration needle will pass through any significant blood vessels. These can be around the vaginal vault and parametrial tissues but also adjacent to the ovaries where the iliac vessels can easily be mistaken for mature follicles if only imaged in one plane. The needle tip needs to be clearly visible to the operator at all times. The initial insertion point of the needle through the vaginal vault should be as lateral as possible to avoid possible damage to the ureters and ovarian blood vessels. It is frequently not possible to identify the ureters on a transvaginal scan during the procedure, so a detailed awareness of anatomy is crucial.

Where possible avoid drainage of cystic structures within the ovary, which can lead to ovarian stromal vessel trauma, as well as increasing the risk of infection. Additionally, the use of the transmyometrial route is associated with an inherently higher risk of concomitant vascular injury.

6.2.1 Minor Local Vaginal Bleeding

Minor local vaginal bleeding at the needle puncture site can nearly always be managed by visualisation of the bleed point followed by gentle application of pressure using a sponge forceps and gauze. It is good practice to visualise these sites prior to completing the procedure and transferring the patient back to recovery. Insertion of a suture to the bleed point will effectively deal with the few cases where local pressure does not control bleeding.

6.2.2 Intra-Abdominal Bleeding

Intra-abdominal bleeding is a potentially life-threatening complication, and to this end, all patients should have vital signs monitored throughout and after the TVOR procedure. However, it is important to understand and allow for the fact that some patients will present some hours after the procedure and not necessarily to the same clinical setting. This may relate to the underlying fitness of most patients who are able to compensate very well for significant blood loss that might otherwise manifest sooner. In addition, slow venous blood loss may not be evident during or immediately after TVOR. Patient information sheets must reflect this fact.

Assessment of these patients will involve vital signs, bloods and cross-matching for intervention either laparoscopically or via open surgery. Pre-operative scanning can sometimes reveal significant free fluid in the pouch of Douglas. It is important that surgeons involved in these procedures are experienced in assessing post-IVF ovaries, which do look 'abnormal' to the inexperienced eye, and can lead to inappropriate and damaging surgical intervention. Damage to a larger vessel should lead to the involvement of the on-call vascular team. In these cases, laparotomy may ultimately be required.

6.3 Empty Follicle Syndrome

The clinical scenario of failure to retrieve any oocytes from apparently normal-looking mature follicles after progression through an optimal IVF stimulation cycle is extremely distressing for patients and also for staff involved in the TVOR procedure. Fortunately, it is relatively rare, occurring in approximately 0.5–2% of IVF cycles [5].

The final maturation process in an IVF cycle involves administration of either exogenous human chorionic gonadotropin (hCG) or use of a gonadotropin-releasing hormone (GnRH) agonist trigger to stimulate endogenous release of luteinising hormone (LH) from the anterior pituitary. The common pathway after this involves completion of oocyte meiosis and maturation, and also causes connective tissue changes in the stalk adhering the cumulus–oocyte complex to the follicular wall. This allows detachment of the oocyte into the follicular fluid, which then allows aspiration from the follicle during TVOR.

Various factors related to hCG/LH can impact this critical process and lead to failure to retrieve oocytes.

6.3.1 Management

In any TVOR procedure where no oocytes are aspirated from several sequential normal follicles, it is prudent to recheck timing details and correct administration of hCG/agonist. Studies have shown that the earliest ovulation post-hCG administration occurs at between 39 and 41 hours. TVOR is usually timed to occur at 36 hours post-trigger to ensure that premature ovulation has not occurred.

The embryologist may notice a sparsity of granulosa cells in the follicular fluid. A catheter urine specimen may be obtained and a high-sensitivity urine pregnancy test can be performed. After subcutaneous hCG injection, urinary hCG levels have been reported as approximately 350 IU; the lower threshold of urine tests is 25–50 IU. If the test is negative, consider giving a further 10,000 IU of hCG from a different batch and rescheduling the TVOR for 36 hours later.

If a urine pregnancy test is positive, then it maybe that there are issues with the bioavailabilty of that particular batch of hCG. Options to consider in future cycles are the use of urinary-derived hCG rather than recombinant hCG. Another option that may be applicable is to change from a GnRH agonist down-regulated cycle to using a GnRH antagonist cycle, which will then allow use of an agonist trigger to generate a surge of endogenous LH, which may be more effective than exogenous hCG.

It has been suggested that in cases where failure to retrieve oocytes in previous cycle has occurred, measurement of serum hCG 12 hours after retrieval can be reassuring, with levels above 50 mIU/ml being deemed adequate.

In cases where adequate hCG levels are measured and failure also occurs with an endogenous LH trigger, it should be considered that a case of true empty follicle syndrome is diagnosed. This conclusion may also be reached in cases of recurrent failure to retrieve in sequential cycles. Provision of expert counselling and consideration of donor oocyte treatment should be considered.

6.4 Oocyte Aspiration Pump Failure

In the early days of IVF, oocyte retrieval from follicles was often achieved using the negative pressure generated by a simple syringe attached to the TVOR needle. Flushing medium was then introduced back into the follicle by virtue of another pre-filled syringe. This was a relatively simple process, but there was scope for considerable variability in the pressures generated, and this could on occasion cause damage to the oocyte. The development of adjustable pumps to which appropriate tubing is attached allows consistent pressure to be applied, which can also be varied appropriately depending on whether the operator is using a single- or double-lumen aspiration needle. This probably also ensures more comprehensive guaranteed sterility of the tubing/tube system. With modern purpose-built pumps, failure during a procedure is fortunately a rare occurrence, but operators need to be clear on how to deal with this alarming scenario if it does happen.

6.4.1 Management
6.4.1.1 Pump Checks

Prevention of this problem is always preferable to having to deal with a failure during the procedure.

All units should have robust standard operating procedures that ensure validation of aspiration pumps when first used and then at regular intervals. Prior to needle insertion when the tubing is attached to the needle and the proximal end to the pump, the pressure reading should always be checked on the machine and then a test aspiration should always be performed to ensure the closed system is working optimally with flushing medium emerging in to an empty tube promptly after pump activation. Problems noted at this point are often easily corrected by reviewing the connection or kinks in tubing. If the bung is not firmly attached to the tube or the tube is cracked, this will result in a loss of vacuum and failure to aspirate fluid.

6.4.1.2 Tubing Checks

Failure or slow drip of fluid into the tube is a frequently encountered problem during the TVOR procedure. This again can relate to issues with tubing and cracked tubes, which can easily be remedied. It is also worth reviewing the exact position of the needle tip to ensure it is centrally placed within the follicular lumen. Constant visualisation of the needle tip at all times coupled with minimal unnecessary movement should prevent this problem.

6.4.1.3 Needle Blockage

Experienced operators will usually be aware of the position of the needle tip due to tactile feedback on entering follicles, and this allied with visual cues should lead to early suspicion of needle blockage due to stromal tissue or possible congealed blood or endometriotic aspirate. At this point, an attempt can be made to clear the lumen of the needle by disconnecting the aspiration system and flushing the needle. The alternative may be withdrawal of the needle and changing this for a new unused one. This should be avoided where possible due to increased risk of complications such as bleeding that are associated with repeated needle insertions.

6.5 Excessive Pain during Oocyte Retrieval

Approaches to pain relief during oocyte retrieval will vary from one centre to another. While some centres use a general anaesthetic, other units use variable degrees of sedation ranging from deep to conscious sedation. In the authors' unit, conscious sedation is practised and has been carefully refined over the years. This involves nurse-administered fentanyl starting usually at a dose of 50 μg given intravenously (IV), with additional doses given throughout the procedure as required to a maximum of 125–150 μg. In addition, the patient self-administers nitrous oxide and the operator administers a local anaesthetic block to the vaginal vault. Prior to the procedure, IV paracetamol is administered.

Although the use of conscious sedation usually works very well and allows the patient and partner to actively engage in the procedure, there are situations when the procedure can be particularly uncomfortable. This should be anticipated in women who have previously had a particularly painful oocyte retrieval, have endometriosis or have high-positioned ovaries. In such cases, units employing conscious sedation protocols should have alternative strategies available.

Often, all that is required is additional support and reassurance throughout the procedure. In addition, in the authors' unit, a higher dose of fentanyl is administered prior to starting the procedure (e.g. 75 μg). Although more frequent administration of additional doses may be used, it is important to time this properly in relationship to the number of oocytes present, or else the operator may find the maximum dose of analgesia has been reached well before the procedure has been completed. It is important in such situations that movements with the needle are minimal and gentle and the number of ovarian punctures are kept to minimum, as this is usually the most painful part of the procedure. In severe situations and where the situation has been anticipated in advance, the procedure may need to be performed under deep sedation or a general anaesthetic.

Finally, it is important to point out that sedation techniques should be developed in liaison with anaesthetic colleges, as what might be a safe regimen in one unit may not be so in another depending on the facilities and proximity to emergency services.

6.6 Incidental Adnexal Pathology

An adnexal cyst may sometimes be large enough to interfere with easy access to the oocytes. For example, an endometrioma may pose a particular challenge. In view of current evidence suggesting that surgery for endometriomas does not improve reproductive outcomes after assisted conception and may in fact have a detrimental effect on the response to stimulation [6, 7], it is not uncommon nowadays to encounter endometriomas at the time of oocyte retrieval. If possible, it is best to avoid penetration of the endometrioma to minimise the risk of infection due to the presence of old blood within the cyst that may act as a good culture medium for micro-organisms [8], although recent studies have been reassuring in this regard [9].

Often, it is necessary to penetrate the endometrioma in order to reach the oocytes. In such cases, it is good practice to administer a prophylactic dose of antibiotics to minimise the risk of subsequent pelvic infection. Another problem encountered with endometriomas is obstruction of the oocyte retrieval needle due to occlusion from passing through the thick fibrous tissue in the cyst wall or occlusion caused by the thick contents of the cyst. If clearing the needle using high-pressure suction is unsuccessful, the needle will need to be changed. Again, large endometriomas detected prior to starting IVF treatment are best addressed prior to starting the IVF cycle in order to facilitate access to the oocytes or indeed to mobilise a high-positioned ovary.

Another common occurrence is the unexpected finding of a hydrosalpinx. Hydrosalpinges can have a significant negative effect on pregnancy rates after IVF treatment and should always, if possible, be addressed before the start of treatment by salpingectomy, salpingostomy or tubal occlusion [10]. However, some hydrosalpinges may be intermittent and therefore missed prior to oocyte retrieval. If the operator has no choice but to penetrate the hydrosalpinx in order to reach the oocytes, then again good practice would be to administer antibiotics to avoid a later potentially serious pelvic infection. It is important to point out that a hydrosalpinx should not be intentionally drained in the belief that this will improve pregnancy rates, as such practice is not supported by evidence and carries an undue risk of infection. The incidental discovery of a hydrosalpinx at the time of oocyte retrieval is best managed by deferring embryo transfer until the hydrosalpinx has been managed surgically by one of the previously mentioned techniques.

References

1. Davis LB, Ginsburg ES. Transmyometrial oocyte retrieval and pregnancy rates. *Fertil Steril* 2004;**81**:320–2. doi: 10.1016/j.fertnstert.2003.06.019

2. Wisanto A, Bollen N, Camus M, et al. Effect of transuterine puncture during transvaginal oocyte retrieval on the results of human in-vitro fertilization. *Hum Reprod* 1989;**4**(7):790–3. doi: 10.1093/oxfordjournals.humrep.a136987

3. Barton SE, Politch JA, Benson CB, Ginsburg ES, Gargiulo AR. Transabdominal follicular aspiration for oocyte retrieval in patients with ovaries inaccessible by transvaginal ultrasound. *Fertil Steril* 2011;**95**(5):1773–6. doi: 10.1016/j.fertnstert.2011.01.006

4. Ludwig AK, Glawatz M, Griesinger G, Diedrich K, Ludwig M. Perioperative and postoperative complications of ultrasound-guided oocyte retrieval: prospective study of more than 1000 oocyte retrievals. *Hum Reprod* 2006;**21**(12):3235–40. doi: 10.1093/humrep/del278

5. Nduwke G, Thornton S, Fishel S, Dowell K, Aloum M. Predicting empty follicle syndrome. *Fertil Steril* 1996;**66**:845–7. doi: 10.1016/S0015-0282(16)58650-6

6. Benschop L, Farquhar C, van der Poel N, Heineman MJ. Interventions for women with endometrioma prior to assisted reproductive technology. *Cochrane Database Syst Rev* 2010;**10**(11):CD008571. doi: 10.1002/14651858.CD008571.pub2

7. Nickkho-Amiry M, Savant R, Majumder K, Edi-O'sagie E, Akhtar M. The effect of surgical management of endometrioma on the IVF/ICSI outcomes when compared with no treatment? A systematic review and meta-analysis. *Arch Gynecol Obstet* 2018;**297**(4):1043–57. doi: 10.1007/s00404-017-4640-1

8. Sharpe K, Karovitch AJ, Claman P, Suh KN. Transvaginal oocyte retrieval for in vitro fertilization complicated by ovarian abscess during pregnancy. *Fertil Steril* 2006;**86**(1):219.e11–13. doi: 10.1016/j.fertnstert.2005.12.045

9. Benaglia L, Busnelli A, Biancardi R, et al. Oocyte retrieval difficulties in women with ovarian endometriomas. *Reprod Biomed Online* 2018;**37**(1):77–84. doi: 10.1016/j.rbmo.2018.03.020

10. Johnson N, van Voorst S, Sowter MC, Strandell A, Mol BW. Surgical treatment for tubal disease in women due to undergo in vitro fertilisation. *Cochrane Database Syst Rev* 2010;**1**:CD002125. doi: 10.1002/14651858.CD002125.pub3

Complications of Oocyte Retrieval

Hajeb Kamali and Valentine Akande

7.1 Introduction

During the fledgling era of in vitro fertilisation (IVF) treatment, oocyte retrieval was performed laparoscopically. However, this relatively invasive procedure necessitated general anaesthesia, significant use of resources and a degree of surgical proficiency from the operator, as well as imposing a period of recovery on the patient. Since its introduction in 1983, the transvaginal ultrasound-guided oocyte retrieval (TVOR) approach has replaced this technique worldwide and is now the gold standard for oocyte retrieval.

Compared with a laparoscopic or abdominal approach, the transvaginal approach has several advantages:

- Improved rates of mature oocyte recovery and fertilisation compared with the laparoscopic approach.
- The use of local anaesthesia and sedation over general anaesthesia.
- Reduced risk of bowel injury.
- Less technically challenging, especially for those trained in transvaginal ultrasound.
- Reduced patient costs.
- Quicker patient recovery post-procedure.
- Reduced post-operative pain.
- Patient preference.

In cases where the ovaries are inaccessible transvaginally, which could be congenital, as a result of an enlarged uterus or adhesions for example, the transabdominal route must be considered. There is a paucity of evidence on complications associated with this approach. A review of 69 cases of transabdominal follicular aspiration reported no serious intraoperative complications and two cases of post-operative infection, one of whom required hospitalisation for parenteral antibiotics [1].

However, inaccessibility of ovaries transvaginally is uncommon, occurring in only 0.4% of cases [1].

Therefore, for the purpose of this chapter, we will focus on risks associated specifically with the transvaginal approach, although many of these will also pertain to the transabdominal approach.

The transvaginal approach is generally considered safe, and rates of complications are low. The latest report from the European Society of Human Reproduction and Embryology (ESHRE) IVF-monitoring Consortium consisting of data on 776,556 treatment cycles found complications reported in 0.17% of cycles [2]. Rates from other large observational studies range from 0.4 to 0.72% [3, 4].

The most commonly reported complications of oocyte retrieval are haemorrhage, pelvic infection, pelvic visceral injury and complications related to sedation or anaesthesia. Rarer complications are often reported in the literature as case reports. Although complications occur infrequently, their consequences should not be underestimated, as deaths have been reported [2].

7.2 Haemorrhage

Arguably, the most common complication of TVOR is vaginal bleeding, occurring to varying degrees in up to 18% of cases [3]. The average blood loss during uncomplicated oocyte retrieval has been estimated to be 72–230 ml and of no clinical significance to most patients [5, 6]. This appears to be unrelated to the number of aspirated follicles, number of eggs collected, pre-ovulatory oestradiol levels and duration of the procedure [5].

Steps that can be taken to minimise this risk include minimising the number of puncture sites and reducing the degree of needle movement within the vaginal wall, especially lateral movement. Adequate haemostasis for bleeding from the vaginal wall can usually be achieved with simple measures such as application of pressure, suturing of the lesion or the use of local haemostatic agents.

Significant intraperitoneal bleeding occurs in 0.06–0.36% of cases [3, 7]. This may occur as a result of direct trauma to the pelvic vasculature or pelvic organs including the ovaries and colon. Cases of iliac vessel injury are usually a result of misinterpretation of iliac vessels in cross-section as ovarian follicles. Early signs of such injury include acute haemodynamic compromise and ultrasound visualisation of real-time fluid accumulation in the pouch of Douglas.

Post-operatively, there may be signs or symptoms of anaemia. Haemodynamic compromise (tachycardia, hypotension, tachypnoea, collapse) should prompt immediate consideration of surgical intervention in the form of an emergency laparoscopy or laparotomy to identify and stem the bleeding. It is crucial to consider, however, that diagnosis may often be delayed. Surgical management is dictated by the cause and source of bleeding, and includes identification and coagulation, as well as application of haemostatic agents to the bleeding point. Angiographic uterine artery embolisation has been reported as a non-surgical approach in cases of haemorrhage secondary to oocyte retrieval [8].

As discussed earlier, the transabdominal route can be considered when the ovaries are inaccessible and high in the pelvis. In cases where the ovaries are fixed posteriorly, it may be necessary to traverse the myometrium (and sometimes even the endometrium) transvaginally. However, one must consider that bleeding risk is increased in such cases, and intrauterine infection and even reduced implantation rates can result if the endometrium is traversed.

Retroperitoneal bleeding has also been reported but may have a later and more indolent presentation. Azem et al. reported on one such case where the initial presentation was with acute abdominal pain and tenesmus immediately following oocyte retrieval [9]. Laparoscopy revealed a retroperitoneal haematoma. Laparotomy was undertaken and the haematoma evacuated, revealing bleeding arising from the mid-sacral vein. This diagnosis should be considered in patients presenting with acute pain following oocyte retrieval in whom there is no evidence of haemoperitoneum.

It is also prudent to consider the increased risk and delayed presentation of haemoperitoneum in patients with an underlying coagulopathy where the interval between oocyte retrieval and presentation may be prolonged. Massive haemoperitoneum has been reported in patients with coagulopathies such as factor XI deficiency, factor VIII deficiency and essential thrombocythaemia [8, 10, 11].

There is, of course, also an associated bleeding risk in patients on anticoagulation therapy with known thrombophilia or a history of thromboembolic events. Mashiach et al. reported two cases of massive delayed intra-abdominal bleeding following oocyte retrieval in such women [12]. In both cases, therapeutic anticoagulation was stopped 16 hours prior to oocyte retrieval, but bleeding occurred more than 2 days later. Therapeutic anticoagulation was recommenced 12 hours post-procedure and the authors propose that this may have been too early. However, as yet no universally agreed guidance exists on the management of patients undergoing oocyte retrieval receiving anticoagulation.

Demonstrating that the structure is round in both the longitudinal and transverse planes by rotating the ultrasound probe prior to puncture will confirm that the structure is a follicle and not a blood vessel (a blood vessel will become elongated as the probe is rotated) and will reduce the risk of vessel injury, as will application of colour Doppler. The operator should always maintain a low threshold for applying these techniques if there is any uncertainty prior to follicular puncture. The pelvis should also be inspected prior to removal of the transvaginal probe in order to exclude significant accumulation of pelvic fluid since the start of the procedure. Specific attention should also be paid to a family history suggestive of coagulopathy or a personal history suggestive of a bleeding tendency in order to identify patients without a pre-existing diagnosis of an underlying coagulopathy. Early and close liaison with a multidisciplinary team including a haematologist in such cases will help to anticipate, individualise and minimise bleeding risk associated with oocyte retrieval.

7.3 Pelvic Infection

The risk of infection is low following oocyte retrieval, with reported rates of 0.04–0.77% for pelvic infection [4, 13] and 0.19% for pelvic abscess [13] from large observational studies. However, the associated risk of hospital admission is high [4]. Several potential mechanisms exist for the development of pelvic infection following oocyte retrieval.

Direct pelvic contamination can occur through puncture of a non-sterile vagina and subsequent transfer of micro-organisms into an ovarian follicle.

The formation of a haematoma or haemorrhagic cyst is likely to further increase the risk of abscess formation, as coagulated blood serves as an ideal culture medium. In fact, commonly encountered vaginal flora have been shown to be found in pelvic abscesses resulting from oocyte retrieval [14].

Entry into a pelvis with chronic infection in women with a history of pelvic inflammatory disease (PID) also increases the risk of pelvic infection following oocyte retrieval. The presence of endometriomas at the time of oocyte retrieval is thought to increase the risk of pelvic abscess, as, again, the cyst content is an ideal culture medium for vaginal flora. Hence, prophylactic antibiotics are encouraged in such cases. In fact, the risk of PID is increased in these patients even if the endometriomas have not been punctured. Surgical drainage (either vaginal or abdominal) should be considered prior to superovulation or oocyte retrieval, and the urge to drain endometriomas at the time of oocyte retrieval should be resisted. In the case of inadvertent puncture, the aspiration needle should be withdrawn and flushed with media. The collecting tube should also be changed before proceeding. A prolonged course of broad-spectrum antibiotics should be considered in this scenario. Rarely, a faecal peritonitis can result from inadvertent bowel injury with the follicular aspiration needle.

There is no consensus regarding the routine administration of prophylactic antibiotics in patients undergoing oocyte retrieval, and evidence is conflicting over the benefits of a blanket policy of antibiotics for all cases. A more selective approach may be prudent in an era of increasing antibiotic resistance, targeting prophylaxis at those with risk factors for pelvic infection such a history of PID, presence of hydrosalpinges, severe endometriosis, ruptured appendicitis or multiple previous pelvic surgeries. Commonly used antibiotic choices include rectal metronidazole, intravenous co-amoxiclav and oral doxycycline.

Other preventative measures for pelvic infection include minimising the number of vaginal penetrations during oocyte retrieval, ensuring meticulous and thorough probe decontamination measures, and checking of the probe cover for defects following oocyte retrieval. Vaginal and forniceal preparation should be undertaken prior to oocyte retrieval, although there is no consensus on the ideal choice of solution. This is generally performed using normal saline rather than an antibacterial agent over concerns of a detrimental effect on pregnancy rate without any reduction in infection risk [15]. Basic hygiene measures should also not be forgotten including hand washing and the use of sterile gloves. As reasonable a sterile field as is realistic should be achieved using sterile drapes over the patient's legs and under the buttocks.

7.4 Injury of Pelvic Structures

Pelvic structures such as ureters, bladder, bowel, pelvic blood vessels and nerves are at risk of injury during TVOR. However, it is difficult to know the true incidence of this, as the majority will remain undetected and resolve spontaneously. Adhesion formation in women with previous PID, multiple surgeries or endometriosis can pose a theoretical risk. In reality, however, the ovaries are often fixed to pelvic peritoneum in such cases, allowing direct access to follicles and reducing the risk of injury to pelvic organs.

Anatomically, the ureters lie in close proximity anterolaterally to the fornices of the upper vagina and are therefore at risk of injury. A history of PID, previous pelvic surgery, the presence of adhesions and endometriosis all increase the risk of ureteral injury as the ureteric course may be altered. Ureteric injury can lead to ureteral obstruction and subsequent hydronephrosis, transection or stricture requiring surgical reimplantation, urine leak into the retroperitoneal space and ureterovaginal fistula. Presentation depends on the site of injury and includes haematuria, dysuria, frequency, abdominal/flank pain, nausea and vomiting, vaginal leakage and fever. A management plan should be made in conjunction with urologists, and frequently involves stent placement and antibiotic therapy.

The internal iliac arteries and their branches are also at risk of injury during oocyte retrieval as a result of their proximity to ovaries. There have been several reports of pseudo-aneurysms of pelvic vessels including internal iliac and obturator arteries [16–18]. Presentation is variable from acute haemorrhagic shock to an incidental finding at an antenatal scan. Management will depend on the diameter and location of the pseudo-aneurysm as well as the haemodynamic status of the patient, and ranges from embolisation in the non-urgent setting to emergency surgery in cases of haemodynamic compromise.

Direct ultrasound visualisation of bowel peristalsis should be used to minimise the risk of inadvertent bowel injury. Transvaginal ultrasound also allows visualisation of the pelvic portion of the ureter, and this should ideally be identified prior to oocyte retrieval to minimise the risk of ureteric injury, especially in patients at risk of alteration of ureteric course and position. The utilisation of colour Doppler and multiplane imaging will aid in differentiation of pelvic vessels from ovarian follicles.

7.5 Vertebral Injury

Bleeding, infection and visceral injury are by far the most common complications of TVOR. However, there have been several reports of bony complications associated with oocyte retrieval. Almog et al. reported on a case of vertebral osteomyelitis following TVOR [19]. Presentation was initially with increased low back pain immediately following the procedure. The patient then re-presented 1 week later with fever and pain in her lower back radiating through her posterior thighs. The diagnosis was eventually made with sequential bone and gallium scans. Kim et al. reported on a patient who presented in her 16th week of pregnancy with low back pain, having undergone TVOR [20]. A lumbar spine magnetic resonance imaging (MRI) scan was suggestive of infectious spondylitis of the L2/L3 vertebrae and spinal biopsy cultured *Staphylococcus aureus*. Spondylodiscitis was also reported by Debusscher et al. following TVOR [21]. Again, the patient presented in the first 24 hours post-procedure with low back pain. An MRI was suggestive of vertebral infiltration at the L5–S1 vertebrae. In this case, however, surgical debridement was required following progression to a peridiscal/vertebral abscess. *Streptococcus faecalis* was isolated. In all of these cases, it is likely that the mechanism of injury involved direct transfer of vaginal micro-organisms to the vertebrae via the tip of the aspiration needle, although haematogenous spread may also have contributed. Although rare, severe or unusual low back pain in anyone having recently undergone TVOR should prompt consideration of such complications.

More rare complications that have been reported in the literature include periumbilical haematoma (Cullen's sign) [22], transient unilateral paresis [23], pelvic tuberculosis [24] and portal vein thrombosis [25], but further discussion of these is outside the scope of this chapter.

Table 7.1. Good practice points for minimising the risk of complications associated with TVOR

Comprehensive pre-operative evaluation including identification of the following risk factors for TVOR:
- History of pelvic inflammatory disease
- Severe endometriosis/endometriomas
- Inaccessible/high ovaries
- Hydrosalpinges
- Previous ruptured appendicitis
- Previous surgery (risk of adhesions and altered ureteric course)
- Bleeding and coagulation defects

Individualised approach to antibiotic therapy in groups at high risk of infection.

Avoidance of repeated ovarian/follicular puncture to reduce risk of intraperitoneal bleeding.

Avoidance of repeated vaginal puncture to reduce risk of pelvic infection.

Dynamic use of ultrasound machine to minimise risk of visceral injury (e.g. use of Doppler flow, identification of bowel peristalsis, ureteric localisation, multiplanar imaging).

Stringent general hygiene measures.

Routine use of World Health Organization checklist or similar before each case.

Early multidisciplinary input when required.

Continued professional development in those undertaking oocyte retrieval:
- Adherence with guidance on safe practices and techniques
- Robust and comprehensive training and supervision
- Regular appraisal

Development of a clinical risk management group within each treating unit where all complications are discussed and adequately investigated.

Adapted from [26].

The good practice points that should be carried out to minimise the risk of complications during TVOR are listed in Table 7.1.

7.6 Summary

Thorough pre-operative evaluation is imperative for all cases of oocyte retrieval in order to identify specific risk factors for complications and allow adaptation of the procedure or technique to minimise this risk. Patients should be adequately counselled about general risks of the procedure but also about their specific individualised risk. Although oocyte retrieval is generally considered safe, all clinicians undertaking oocyte retrieval should have an appreciation of the potential complications associated with the procedure in order to promote early identification and prompt management, thus minimising the associated short- and long-term morbidity for these patients.

References

1. Barton SE, Politch JA, Benson CB, Ginsburg ES, Gargiulo AR. Transabdominal follicular aspiration for oocyte retrieval in patients with ovaries inaccessible by transvaginal ultrasound. *Fertil Steril* 2011;**95**(5):1773–6. doi: 10.1016/j.fertnstert.2011.01.006

2. de Geyter C, Calhaz-Jorge C, Kupka MS, et al. ART in Europe, 2014: results generated from European registries by ESHRE: The European IVF-monitoring Consortium (EIM) for the European Society of Human Reproduction and Embryology (ESHRE). *Hum Reprod* 2018;**33**(9):1586–601. doi: 10.1093/humrep/dey242

3. Siristatidis CS, Vrachnis N, Creatsa M, Maheshwari A, Bhattacharya S. In vitro maturation in subfertile women with polycystic ovarian syndrome undergoing assisted reproduction. *Cochrane Database Syst Rev* 2013;**10**: CD006606. doi: 10.1002/14651858.CD006606.pub3

4. Levi-Setti PE, Cirillo F, Scolaro V, et al. Appraisal of clinical complications after 23,827 oocyte retrievals in a large assisted reproductive technology program. *Fertil Steril* 2018;**109**(6):1038–43. doi: 10.1016/j.fertnstert.2018.02.002

5. Dessole S, Rubattu G, Ambrosini G, et al. Blood loss following noncomplicated transvaginal oocyte retrieval for in vitro fertilization. *Fertil Steril* 2001;**76**(1):205–6. doi: 10.1016/s0015-0282(01)01858-1

6. Ragni G, Scarduelli C, Calanna G, et al. Blood loss during transvaginal oocyte retrieval.

Gynecol Obstet Invest 2009;**67**(1):32–5. doi: 10.1159/000158649

7. Aragona C, Mohamed MA, Espinola MSB, et al. Clinical complications after transvaginal oocyte retrieval in 7,098 IVF cycles. *Fertil Steril* 2011;**95**(1):293–4. doi: 10.1016/j.fertnstert.2010.07.1054

8. Kart C, Guven S, Aran T, Dinc H. Life-threatening intraabdominal bleeding after oocyte retrieval successfully managed with angiographic embolization. *Fertil Steril* 2011;**96**(2):e99–102. doi: 10.1016/j.fertnstert.2011.05.086

9. Azem F, Wolf Y, Botchan A, et al. Massive retroperitoneal bleeding: a complication of transvaginal ultrasonography-guided oocyte retrieval for in vitro fertilization–embryo transfer. *Fertil Steril* 2000;**74**(2):405–6. doi: 10.1016/s0015-0282(00)00637-3

10. Battaglia C., Regnani G., Giulini S., et al. Severe intraabdominal bleeding after transvaginal oocyte retrieval for IVF-ET and coagulation factor XI deficiency: a case report. *J Assist Reprod Genet* 2001;**18**(3):178–81. doi: 10.1023/a:1009468222103

11. El-Shawarby SA, Margara RA, Trew GH, Laffan MA, Lavery SA. Thrombocythemia and hemoperitoneum after transvaginal oocyte retrieval for in vitro fertilization. *Fertil Steril* 2004;**82**(3):735–7. doi: 10.1016/j.fertnstert.2004.01.044

12. Mashiach R, Stockheim D, Zolti M, Orvieto R. Delayed intra-abdominal bleeding following trans-vaginal ultrasonography guided oocyte retrieval for in vitro fertilization in patients at risk for thrombo-embolic events under

anticoagulant therapy. *F1000Research* 2013;**2**:189. doi: 10.12688/f1000research.2-189.v2

13. Özaltın S, Kumbasar S, Savan K. Evaluation of complications developing during and after transvaginal ultrasound-guided oocyte retrieval. *Ginekol Pol* 2018;**89**(1):1–6. doi: 10.5603/GP.a2018.0001

14. Bennett SJ, Waterstone JJ, Cheng WC, Parsons J. Complications of transvaginal ultrasound-directed follicle aspiration: a review of 2670 consecutive procedures. *J Assist Reprod Genet* 1993;**10**(1):72–7. doi: 10.1007/BF01204444

15. van Os HC, Drogendijk AC, Fetter WPF, Heijtink RA, Zeilmaker GH. The influence of contamination of culture medium with hepatitis B virus on the outcome of in vitro fertilization pregnancies. *Am J Obstet Gynecol* 1991;**165**(1):152–9. doi: 10.1016/0002-9378(91)90244-l

16. Bolster F, Mocanu E, Geoghegan T, Lawler L. Transvaginal oocyte retrieval complicated by life-threatening obturator artery haemorrhage and managed by a vessel-preserving technique. *Ulster Med J* 2014;**83**(3):146.

17. Pappin C, Plant G. A pelvic pseudoaneurysm (a rare complication of oocyte retrieval for IVF) treated by arterial embolization. *Hum Fertil* 2006;**9**(3):153–5. doi: 10.1080/14647270600595952

18. Bozdag G, Basaran A, Cil B, Esinler İ, Yarali H. An oocyte pick-up procedure complicated with pseudoaneurysm of the internal iliac artery. *Fertil Steril*

2008;**90**(5):2004.e11–13. doi: 10.1016/j.fertnstert.2008.02.010

19. Almog B, Rimon E, Yovel I, et al. Vertebral osteomyelitis: a rare complication of transvaginal ultrasound-guided oocyte retrieval. *Fertil Steril* 2000;**73** (6):1250–2. doi: 10.1016/s0015-0282(00)00538-0

20. Kim HH, Yun NR., Kim DM, Kim SA. Successful delivery following staphylococcus aureus bacteremia after in vitro fertilization and embryo transfer. *Chonnam Med J* 2015;**51**(1):47–9. doi: 10.4068/cmj.2015.51.1.47

21. Debusscher F, Troussel S, van Innis F, Holemans X. Spondylodiscitis after transvaginal oocyte retrieval for in vitro fertilisation. *Acta Orthop Belg* 2005;**71**(2):249–51.

22. Bentov Y, Levitas E, Silberstein T, Potashnik G. Cullen's sign following ultrasound-guided transvaginal oocyte retrieval. *Fertil Steril* 2006;**85** (1):227.e9–12. doi: 10.1016/j.fertnstert.2005.06.054

23. van Eenige MM, Scheele F, van Haaften M, Westrate W, Jansen CAM. A case of a neurological complication after transvaginal oocyte retrieval. *J Assist Reprod Genet* 1997;**14**(1):21–2. doi: 10.1007/BF02765746

24. Annamraju H, Ganapathy R, Webb B. Pelvic tuberculosis reactivated by in vitro fertilization egg collection? *Fertil Steril* 2008;**90**(5):2003.e1–3. doi: 10.1016/j.fertnstert.2008.02.147

25. Mmbaga N, Torrealday S, McCarthy S, Rackow BW. Acute portal vein thrombosis complicating in vitro fertilization. *Fertil Steril* 2012;**98**(6):1470–3. doi: 10.1016/j.fertnstert.2012.08.010

26. El-Shawarby SA, Margara RA, Trew GH, Lavery SA. A review of complications following transvaginal oocyte retrieval for in-vitro fertilization. *Hum Fertil* 2004;**7**(2):127–33. doi: 10.1080/14647270410001699081

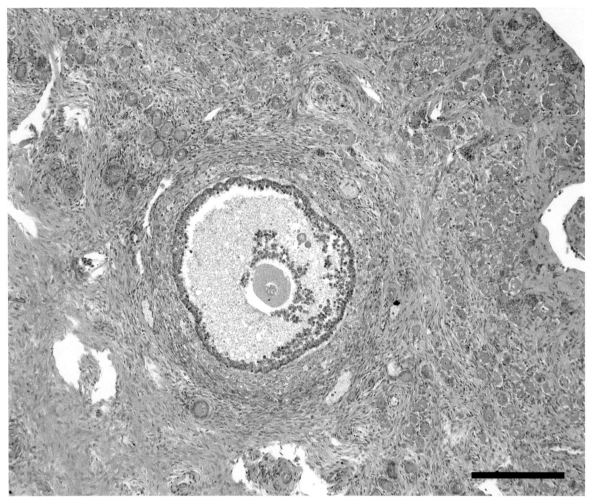

Figure 1.1 The human neonatal ovary. Numerous primordial follicles are embedded in the stroma, and a small antral follicle measuring approximately 400 μm in diameter is evident (centre). Although the antral follicle appears well developed, it is destined to undergo atresia due to insufficient levels of gonadotrophins in early life. Scale bar = 200 μm. A black and white version of this figure will appear in some formats. For the colour version, refer to the plate section. Image kindly provided by Dr Suzannah Williams and Briet Bjarkadottir (University of Oxford).

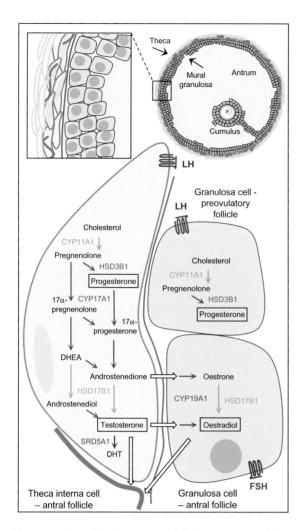

Figure 1.2 Steroid synthesis in antral follicles. During antral follicle development, luteinising hormone (LH) binds to the LH receptor on theca cells, which regulates the expression and activity of key steroidogenic enzymes, allowing the modification of cholesterol into androgens. Testosterone and androstenedione diffuse across the basement membrane where they are converted to oestrogens through the activity of aromatase (CYP19A1), which is regulated by follicle-stimulating hormone (FSH) signalling in granulosa cells. In pre-ovulatory follicles, LH receptor is also expressed in granulosa cells to further amplify progesterone synthesis. Note: steroidogenic enzymes are presented as protein symbols (refer to main text for protein name) with corresponding coloured arrows indicating enzyme activity. A black and white version of this figure will appear in some formats. For the colour version, refer to the plate section.

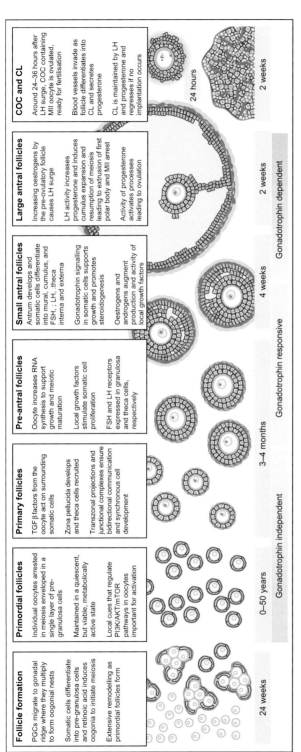

Follicle formation	Primordial follicles	Primary follicles	Pre-antral follicles	Small antral follicles	Large antral follicles	COC and CL
PGCs migrate to gonadal ridge where they multiply to form oogonial nests	Individual oocytes arrested in meiosis enveloped in a single layer of pre-granulosa cells	TGFβ factors from the oocyte act on surrounding somatic cells	Oocyte increases RNA synthesis to support growth and meiotic maturation	Antrum develops and somatic cells differentiate into mural, cumulus, and FSH, ; LH, .theca interna and externa	Increasing oestrogens by the pre-ovulatory follicle causes LH surge	Around 24–36 hours after LH surge. COC containing MII oocyte is ovulated, ready for fertilisation
Somatic cells differentiate into pre-granulosa cells and retinoic acid induces oogonia to initiate meiosis	Maintained in a quiescent, but viable, metabolically active state	Zona pellucida develops and theca cells recruited	Local growth factors stimulate somatic cell proliferation	Gonadotrophin signalling in somatic cells supports growth and promotes steroidogenesis	LH activity increases progesterone and induces cumulus expansion and resumption of meiosis leading to extrusion of first polar body and MII arrest	Blood vessels invade as follicle differentiates into CL and secretes progesterone
Extensive remodelling as primordial follicles form	Local cues that regulate PI3K/AKT/mTOR pathways in oocytes important for activation	Transzonal projections and junctional complexes ensure bidirectional communication and synchronous cell development	FSH and LH receptors expressed in granulosa and theca cells, respectively	Oestrogens and androgens augment production and activity of local growth factors	Activity of progesterone activates processes leading to ovulation	CL is maintained by LH and progesterone and regresses if no implantation occurs

24 weeks	0–50 years	3–4 months		4 weeks	2 weeks	24 hours / 2 weeks
Gonadotrophin independent	Gonadotrophin independent		Gonadotrophin responsive	Gonadotrophin dependent		

Figure 1.3 Summary of germ cell development from follicle formation to ovulation. Key stage-specific events are indicated in the text boxes. CL, corpus luteum; FSH, follicle-stimulating hormone; LH, luteinising hormone; MII, metaphase II. A black and white version of this figure will appear in some formats. For the colour version, refer to the plate section.

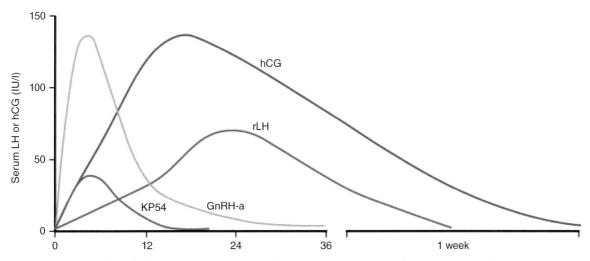

Figure 2.1 Serum profiles of inductors of oocyte maturation. The x-axis shows time (hours) after administration. hCG, human chorionic gonadotropin; rLH, recombinant luteinising hormone; GnRH-a, gonadotropin-releasing hormone antagonist; KP54, kisspeptin-54. A black and white version of this figure will appear in some formats. For the colour version, refer to the plate section. Reproduced from Abbara et al. [14].

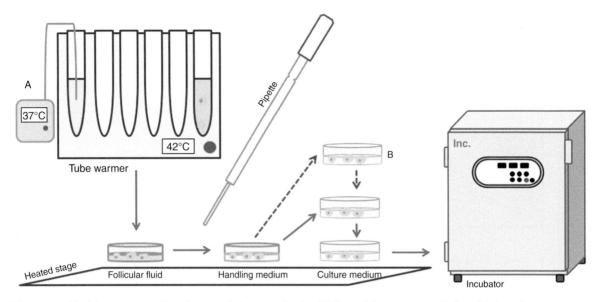

Figure 10.1 The laboratory processing of oocytes during egg collection. (A) External thermometer probe for validating tube warmer temperature setting. (B) Inclusion of an extra wash step in culture medium. A black and white version of this figure will appear in some formats. For the colour version, refer to the plate section.

Likelihood	Consequence				
	Insignificant (1)	Minor (2)	Moderate (3)	Major (4)	Catastrophic (5)
Rare (1)	1	2	3	4	5
Unlikely (2)	2	4	6	8	10
Possible (3)	3	6	9	12	15
Likely (4)	4	8	12	16	20
Almost certain (5)	5	10	15	20	25

Figure 10.2 Risk rating during a risk assessment. A black and white version of this figure will appear in some formats. For the colour version, refer to the plate section.

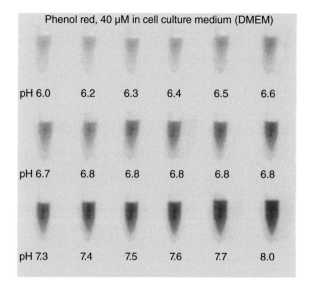

Phenol red, 40 µM in cell culture medium (DMEM)

pH 6.0	6.2	6.3	6.4	6.5	6.6
pH 6.7	6.8	6.8	6.8	6.8	6.8
pH 7.3	7.4	7.5	7.6	7.7	8.0

Figure 12.3 Phenol red, showing the different colours at acid, neutral and alkaline conditions. DMEM, Dulbecco's modified Eagle's medium. Image modified from Wikipedia. A black and white version of this figure will appear in some formats. For the colour version, refer to the plate section.

The Transport IVF Process

1 Satellite clinic

In transport IVF, most of the direct interaction with patients, from ovarian stimulation to ultrasound-guided follicular fluid aspiration, is conducted at a satellite clinic.

2 Transportation

The follicular aspirates are then transported under strictly controlled conditions to an IVF laboratory.

3 Fertilisation occurs

Fertilisation of embryos is conducted in the IVF laboratory.

4 Returned to clinic

The fertilised embryos are then returned to the satellite clinic for implantation.

Figure 12.5 Flow diagram showing how transport IVF programmes work. Modified from Bridge Clinic, www.thebridgeclinic.com. A black and white version of this figure will appear in some formats. For the colour version, refer to the plate section.

The Nurse's Role during Oocyte Retrieval

Alison McTavish

8.1 Introduction

The role of the nurse is to provide a holistic approach to all aspects of fertility care by addressing the physical, mental and emotional health of patients throughout their treatment. Within a fertility setting, the majority of patients are seen as couples, which brings another dimension when Nurses providing care to each individual need to be aware of the impact of infertility on each person and also on the couples' relationship. The nursing team is made up of staff who bring different ranges of knowledge, skills and experience to the team; these can include:

- Healthcare support workers (HCSW) who are trained locally.
- Nursing associates, who have undertaken nationally recognised training and can bridge the gap between HCSWs and trained registered nurses.
- Registered nurses, who have undertaken 3 years of training and meet the standards set by the Nursing and Midwifery Council (NMC).
- Registered midwives, who have undertaken 3 years of training, or have trained as nurses and undertaken a further 18 months of training in midwifery and meet the standards set by the NMC.

The NMC Code (2015), which all registered nurses must adhere to, has four core values all of which should be utilised during oocyte retrieval [1]:

- *Prioritising people* by treating the person having the procedure with dignity, listening to their preferences and concerns, acting in their best interests and respecting everyone's right to privacy and confidentiality.
- *Practising effectively* by ensuring practice is in line with the best available evidence, communicating clearly, working co-operatively, and sharing skills, knowledge and experience for the benefit of the patient undergoing the surgical

procedure. This includes keeping clear and accurate records.

- *Preserving safety* by working within the limits of competence and acting as the patient's advocate by raising concerns immediately if the patient appears vulnerable or at risk and needs extra support and protection. Nurses should advise on and can prescribe, supply, dispense or administer medicines depending on their training and competence.
- *Promoting professionalism and trust.* This is a cornerstone of professional practice and requires fertility nurses to uphold the reputation of the profession always and provide leadership to ensure individual well-being is protected, while improving an individual's experiences of the healthcare system.

To be able to present an overview of the roles nurses undertake during oocyte retrieval, I sent a questionnaire to 32 centres licensed by the Human Fertilisation and Embryology Authority (HFEA) in the UK. Throughout this chapter, I will include the feedback from the questionnaire regarding the ways in which nursing staff are involved in this procedure varies hugely from centre to centre.

8.2 Planning Oocyte Retrieval

When the decision is made to go ahead and plan oocyte retrieval, it is usually the nursing staff who relay the important information to the patient. The information can be given via telephone, text or using a patient app or a portal to an electronic database. Whichever way the information is relayed to the patient, it must be clear when to stop the endogenous gonadotrophins, agonist or antagonist medication, and when to take the trigger injection.

Patients must also be advised when to stop eating and drinking, and in some centres they will also be advised to take paracetamol and ibuprofen 1 hour before the procedure with a few sips of water. The other instructions given relate to no perfumed products being worn, no cosmetics (especially no nail varnish) and no jewellery other than wedding rings. These instructions are provided to partners if they wish to accompany the patient into the procedure room. When providing the information, the nursing staff can also answer any questions that the patients may have to allay any anxiety prior to the procedure.

Section 15.1 of the 9th edition of the HFEA Code of Practice states that centres should have documented procedures for oocyte retrieval, sedation, resuscitation, and prevention and management of ovarian hyperstimulation syndrome [2]. Each centre should have their own standard operating procedure (SOP), which should be validated and audited regularly to ensure that patients are treated safely.

8.3 Sperm Sample

If a fresh sperm sample is produced at home, the nursing staff should ensure as far as possible that the identity of the sperm provider is confirmed: the person providing the sample must confirm that they produced the sample, record the date and time of production, and check that the receptacle is appropriate, is clearly labelled and has not been interfered with (see section 18.12 in [2]). If the sample is to be produced on site, nursing staff must ensure that the person producing the sample and the identification on the semen pot match, and this needs to be double witnessed and recorded in the medical records.

8.4 Documented Procedures: Oocyte Retrieval

Nursing staff should ensure that the SOP for oocyte retrieval clearly states what equipment should be available and how it should be set up. The nursing team are responsible for ensuring the sterility of the equipment and also that all equipment is working and there are no concerns. The SOP should also document the process for welcoming and identifying both the patient and their partner or person accompanying patient to provide support throughout the procedure.

The pre-anaesthetic checklist must be completed, ensuring that the patient and, if present, their partner are prepared for theatre. It is important to record when the trigger medication was taken, as there have been occasions when it has not been taken at the correct

time which must be 34–36 hours before oocyte retrieval. If it has not been taken or taken only 12 hours before the patient arrived at the centre, the patient will be sent home and the procedure rescheduled. If it was taken more than 36 hours earlier, an ultrasound scan could be carried out to assess whether the follicles are still there or whether ovulation has occurred, in which case the procedure cannot be undertaken.

All nursing staff must ensure patient safety during oocyte retrieval. The surgical pause/huddle prior to the theatre list commencing should be attended by all involved in the process and led by the person undertaking the procedure, which in some centres could be a nurse. The theatre team should be clear about their roles and be aware of any medical needs, allergy status and patient history; all team members should be aware of the procedure to be undertaken and are clear of who is leading the briefing, as well as any critical information such as language barriers or disability.

8.5 Sedation

A recent Cochrane review on pain relief for women undergoing oocyte retrieval, which included 24 randomised controlled trials (3,160 women in total) concluded that: 'The evidence does not support one particular method or technique over another in providing effective conscious sedation and analgesia for pain relief during and after oocyte retrieval' [3].

This is reflected in the responses to the questionnaire, which revealed that 84% (27) centres used intravenous sedation alone, while the remaining 16% (five) used general anaesthetic for oocyte recovery. Regardless of the sedation or anaesthetic used, nursing staff must be competent in caring for the patient throughout the procedure and act as an advocate when needed.

8.6 World Health Organization (WHO) Surgical Pathway

Patients should arrive around 45 minutes before the procedure to meet with the nurse and anaesthetist or sedation provider. The surgical pathway should include all steps listed in the WHO Surgical Safety Checklist document [4] and be followed throughout any procedure undertaken that requires anaesthesia, conscious sedation or local anaesthetics.

Before the induction of sedation or anaesthesia, the nurse and anaesthetist/seditionist should carry out the following:

- Verbally confirm the patient's identity.
- Explain what is going to happen throughout the procedure.
- Ensure all consents are in place and have been accurately completed.
- Check with the patient if they have a known allergy.
- Check with the patient if they have any difficulty with airway or aspiration risk.

The other issues on the checklist are regarding marking the site of the operation with a permanent marker, which is not applicable for oocyte retrieval, and to assess the risk of blood loss and be proactive if the risk of blood loss is greater than 500 ml. This process is usually undertaken in the day ward/pre-theatre area.

In the theatre setting, the nurse, anaesthetist and surgeon should confirm that all team members have introduced themselves by name and role, and in turn the patient should confirm their name. Embryologists also join the patient and clinical staff to witness the patient identification.

Some centres may use antibiotic prophylaxis, which should be recorded; however, there is some evidence that only patients with a history of endometriosis, pelvic inflammatory disease, ruptured appendicitis or multiple prior pelvic surgeries should be given antibiotics [5].

8.7 Resuscitation Equipment

Before any theatre list, nursing staff should check and record that they have checked the emergency resuscitation equipment and also the expiry date on the emergency medicines pack. The Misuse of Drugs Act 1971 places controls on certain medicines which are commonly called controlled drugs that are used during oocyte retrieval [6]. The National Institute for Health and Care Excellence (NICE) guideline provides information regarding the processes for using and managing controlled drugs safely in all National Health Service (NHS) settings except care homes [7].

Nursing staff must work within the *Professional Guidance on the Administration of Medicines in Healthcare Settings*, which has been produced by the Royal Pharmaceutical Society and the Royal College of Nursing (RCN) [8]. Nurses who administer medicines must be appropriately trained, assessed as competent, and meet relevant professional and regulatory standards and guidance.

8.8 Survey of Nurses Undertaking Pre-procedure Checklist

Part of the survey was to ask which members of the nursing team were involved in the oocyte retrieval process and the answers provided made it clear that the nurse's role is varied throughout the process. Nurses welcomed the patient to the pre-theatre area and undertook the pre-procedure checklist in 27 (84%) of the 32 responses. In two centres, patients were welcomed by HCSWs, and in three centres, patients went to the theatre area where the pre-procedure checklist was undertaken by the nurse sedationist (two centres) or anaesthetist (one centre).

8.9 Trans People Undergoing Oocyte Retrieval

In January 2016, the House of Commons Women and Equalities Select Committee published its Transgender Equality report, which found that: 'Trans people encounter significant problems in using general NHS services, due to the attitude of some clinicians and other staff who lack knowledge and understanding – and in some cases are prejudiced. The NHS is failing to ensure zero tolerance of transphobic behaviour' [9].

In response to this, the RCN produced guidance on fair care for trans people to ensure that nursing staff help to create a safe and welcoming environment [10].

However, a study on the experiences of transgender men should remind all involved in the procedure of the feelings voiced in this paper, which should underpin the nursing care provided [11]:

> Nakedness and pelvic examinations also functioned as a sort of revealing act. From being seen as a man before the examination, undressing and climbing up into the examination chair exposed them to being seen as women. This also manifested itself when health care professionals used the wrong pronoun when talking about them with others in the room. In addition, the use of gender-specific words, such as 'egg', 'vagina', 'ovaries' and 'uterus', created irritation and distress, reminding them of their gender incongruence/dysphoria as well as confirming that others saw them as a woman.
>
> …The participants coped with stress and negative feelings by focusing on the purpose of the FP [fertility preservation], that is, their ability to have genetically related children in the future. They repeatedly reminded themselves about this during the FP procedures.

Fertility nurses should ensure that they are giving clear information, support and guidance to meet the individual needs of both patient and partner throughout the procedure.

8.10 Undergoing Oocyte Retrieval for Fertility Preservation

Women diagnosed with cancer or any other medical condition that will require treatment that has the potential to make them sterile in the future have to make time-pressured decisions regarding fertility preservation. This patient group must be given as much information as possible; however, the time constraints mean that decisions have to be made fairly quickly and, once decided, treatment usually starts as soon as possible. At the time of oocyte retrieval, nursing staff must ensure that all involved in the procedure are aware of the purpose of this procedure, as it is often undertaken on a routine oocyte retrieval theatre list. However, the patient workup is very different to the infertile patient who has had many months if not years of attending the fertility services prior to having in vitro fertilisation treatment.

In some situations, the age of the patient, or the fact that her mum is accompanying her, acts as a reminder to all in the theatre of the circumstances. The NMC Core value of 'prioritising people' as mentioned earlier relates to treating the person having the procedure with dignity and listening to their preferences and concerns, and should ensure that the procedure is atraumatic as possible.

8.11 The Oocyte Retrieval Process

There are some centres where nurses perform oocyte retrieval; however, in other centres, fertility nurses are not involved in the oocyte retrieval process as this procedure is undertaken within the theatre suite.

All medical and nursing staff who undertake oocyte retrieval must make sure that patients are fully informed about what to expect during the procedure, and that they remain comfortable and safe while as many mature eggs as possible are retrieved using vaginal ultrasound.

The *RCN Education and Career Progression Framework for Fertility Nursing* published in March 2019 provides an overview of the oocyte retrieval process by listing the areas of knowledge required by nurses involved in this procedure as follows [12]:

- *Prepare patient for theatre* in accordance with the WHO Surgical Safety Checklist and also local SOPs, which should be evidence based and referenced. Of the centres I surveyed, 20/32 (62.5%) schedule the retrievals at 20-minute intervals, 10/32 (33%) at 45-minute intervals and 2/32 (6.25%) at 40-minute intervals. Patients should be advised as to how long the procedure could take.
- *Provide assistance during the procedure where required.* The roles undertaken by the nurse according to the feedback from the questionnaire are: assisting in theatre by flushing and changing tubes, taking the tubes of follicular fluid to the embryologists and taking the flushing media to the operator, setting up the scan machine for needle guide, and preparing a trolley with a sterile field for equipment and instruments.

The majority of the centres surveyed reported that it was usually an NMC registered nurse who was 'flooring' and transferring the tubes. In some centres, the HCSW is responsible for the safe collection of follicular fluid. The HCSW works with the person undertaking the oocyte retrieval by collecting the follicular fluid and changing the tubes when advised, with another HCSW transferring the tubes to the heated block.

A recent Cochrane review on follicular flushing during oocyte retrieval found that the 'data suggests little or no difference between follicular flushing and aspiration alone with respect to oocyte yield, total embryo numbers, or number of cryopreserved embryos...and makes no difference in the clinical pregnancy rates' [13]. In keeping with the NMC Code, nurses must 'practice effectively by ensuring practice is in line with the best available evidence' and should therefore challenge any practices that do not reflect the most up-to-date evidence.

8.12 Assessing Patient Well-Being

Throughout the procedure, nursing staff will monitor the patient's vital signs and many will complete the National Early Warning Score (NEWS) chart, which improves the detection and response to clinical deterioration and is a key element of patient safety and improving patient outcomes [14]. The chart has six physiological parameters:

1. Respiratory rate.
2. Oxygen saturation.

3. Temperature.
4. Systolic blood pressure.
5. Pulse rate.
6. Level of consciousness (this will be impaired in patients who have had recent sedation or are receiving opioid analgesia, which should be taken into consideration in assessment).

Nursing staff must also act as the patient's advocate, which requires responding when the patient expresses how she is coping with the procedure, as well as reacting to the vital sign recordings. Prior to and throughout the procedure, the nurse can act as a witness for controlled drug medication dispensing and dosing.

8.13 Risks of Oocyte Retrieval Procedure

As with all surgical procedures, there are potential risks that nursing staff must be prepared for at any time throughout the procedure. The procedure requires a needle to be pushed through the vaginal wall into the ovary, and a number of other organs and sensitive tissues lie nearby. The internal iliac artery runs past the ovary, as does the ureter. The nursing staff in attendance must be aware of their role should an emergency situation occur, which may require vascular surgeon input.

Another complication of oocyte recovery is infection, and therefore nursing staff must ensure that trolleys are set up using aseptic techniques. All healthcare professionals have a responsibility to adhere to local and national infection control policies. Standard infection control precautions need to be applied, and the recommendations are divided into five interventions, all of which apply to the oocyte retrieval process:

1. *Hospital/clinic environment.* Record that the area has been cleaned with appropriate non-toxic materials.
2. *Hand hygiene.* The WHO Guidelines on Hand Hygiene in Health Care: A Summary is an excellent document, which was published due to the healthcare-associated infections that affect hundreds of millions of patients worldwide every year [15]. It includes indications as to when hand washing should be undertaken, and techniques for washing hands using soap and water or alcohol-based formulation are clearly illustrated, as is

surgical hand preparation and the use and handling of gloves. The WHO 'My five moments for hand hygiene' within this document state that hand hygiene should occur:

1. Before touching a patient.
2. Before a clean/aseptic procedure.
3. After body fluid exposure risk.
4. After touching a patient.
5. After touching patient surroundings.

3. *Personal protective equipment.* Plastic aprons should be worn where there is a possibility or a risk of contact with blood or body fluids. Theatre scrubs should always be clean and uncontaminated and changed daily. Disposable and single-use-only caps should be worn to prevent hair from falling onto a sterile surface, but face masks do not need to be used for oocyte retrieval procedures. Special footwear worn in theatres is for that use only and must be cleaned after every use and/or session.
4. *Safe use and disposal of sharps.* Sharps injuries are one of the most common types of injury to be reported to occupational health services by healthcare staff.
5. *Principles of asepsis.* Measures to prevent an infection from entering a wound are undertaken within the theatre/procedure room. These should include hand washing (scrubbing), wearing appropriate clothing specifically for undertaking procedures and using sterile operating instruments (e.g. speculum), which should be opened onto a sterile field.

8.14 Post-operative Care

Nursing staff should be able to diagnose and manage post-operative complications. Following the procedure, vital signs recorded (pulse, respiration rate and blood pressure) should be monitored as, while oocyte retrieval is seen as a minor surgical procedure and the majority of women undergoing it are young and healthy, there are risks associated, and careful post-operative management is essential. When assessing the post-operative patient, the NEWS chart should be used. Any blood loss per vagina must also be checked and recorded – this should be nil. The patient should also be observed for signs of internal haemorrhage, shock, and the effects of analgesia and anaesthetic. Observations should be recorded as requested by the operator until stable prior to being discharged.

8.15 Pre-discharge

If all vital signs are within normal parameters and there are no visible signs of vaginal bleeding, the patient can eat and drink usually within half an hour post-procedure. The intravenous cannula that was used to administer medication can be removed and the patient is encouraged to sit up and walk to the toilet. The use of analgesia medication post-procedure for pain relief and luteal-phase support, if appropriate, should be discussed, and written information should also be provided.

Nursing staff must advise the patient and partner of the out-of-hours contact details, which could include providing an emergency mobile number should this be required. In some centres, patients are seen by embryologists prior to discharge to discuss the number and quality of oocytes retrieved, the quality of the semen sample and to confirm the actual process that is going to be used in the laboratory. In cases of potential cryopreservation of all gametes or embryos, patients may also be reviewed by medical staff prior to discharge.

The patient may be discharged when she feels well. Should the patient require further monitoring, or an overnight stay, admission should be arranged.

The nurse's role does not stop with the discharge of the patient as it is good practice to contact the patient in the days following oocyte retrieval to offer support and ensure any pain is being controlled and so the patient can ask any questions to help reduce anxiety.

8.16 Summary

The nurse's role during oocyte recovery is a continuation of the nursing care provided throughout the patient's fertility treatment. Nurses undertake a leadership role in planning the oocyte retrieval, and a caring and clinical role throughout the surgical processes. The nurse's role is varied but always remains as an advocate for patient well-being. Nurses are aware that every interaction they have with patients and partners throughout the oocyte recovery process can have an impact on their lives and therefore undertake this role in an emotionally intelligent way to provide the best care for each and every patient.

References

1. Nursing and Midwifery Council (NMC). *The Code: Professional Standards of Practice and Behaviour for Nurses, Midwives and Nursing Associates.* London: NMC, 2015. Available from: www.nmc.org.uk/standards/code/

2. Human Fertilisation and Embryology Authority (HEFA). *Code of Practice*, 9th ed. London: HEFA, 2018. Available from: https://portal.hfea.gov.uk/knowledge-base/read-the-code-of-practice/

3. Kwan I, Wang R, Pearce E, Bhattacharya S. Pain relief for women undergoing oocyte retrieval for assisted reproduction. *Cochrane Database Syst Rev* 2018;**5**:CD004829. doi: 10.1002/14651858.CD004829.pub4

4. World Health Organization (WHO). *WHO Surgical Safety Checklist.* Geneva: WHO, 2009. Available from: www.who.int/teams/integrated-health-services/patient-safety/research/safe-surgery/tool-and-resources

5. Pereira N, Hutchinson AP, Lekovich JP, Hobeika E, Elias RT. Antibiotic Prophylaxis for gynecologic procedures prior to and during the utilization of assisted reproductive technologies: a systematic review. *J Pathog* 2016;**2016**: 4698314. doi: 10.1155/2016/4698314

6. The Misuse of Drugs Act 1971. Available from: www.legislation.gov.uk/ukpga/1971/38/contents

7. National Institute for Health and Care Excellence (NICE). *Controlled Drugs: Safe Use and Management.* NICE guideline NG46. London: NICE, 2016. Available from: www.nice.org.uk/guidance/ng46

8. Royal Pharmaceutical Society (RPS)/Royal College of Nursing (RCN). *Professional Guidance on the Administration of Medicines in Healthcare Settings.* London: RPS/RCN, 2019. Available from: www.rcn.org.uk/clinical-topics/medicines-management/professional-resources

9. House of Commons Women and Equalities Select Committee. *Transgender Equality.* London: House of Commons, 2016. https://publications.parliament.uk/pa/cm201516/cmselect/cmwomeq/390/390.pdf

10. Royal College of Nursing (RCN). *Fair Care for Trans People.* London: RCN, 2016.

11. Armuand G, Dhejne C, Olofsson JI, Rodriguez-Wallberg KA. Transgender men's experiences of fertility preservation: a qualitative study. *Hum Reprod* 2017;**32**

(2):383–90. doi: 10.1093/humrep/dew323.

12. Royal College of Nursing (RCN). *An RCN Education and Career Progression Framework for Fertility Nursing*. London, RCN, 2021. Available from: www.rcn.org.uk/professional-development/publications/rcn-education-and-career-progression-framework-for-fertility-nursing-009-926-uk-pub

13. Georgiou EX, Melo P, Brown J, Granne IE, Cochrane Gynaecology and Fertility Group. Follicular flushing during oocyte retrieval in assisted reproductive techniques. *Cochrane Database Syst Rev* 2018; 4:CD004634. doi: 10.1002/14651858.CD004634.pub3

14. Royal College of Physicians. National Early Warning Score (NEWS) 2: standardising the assessment of acute-illness severity in the NHS. www.rcplondon.ac.uk/projects/outputs/national-early-warning-score-news-2

15. World Health Organization (WHO), WHO Patient Safety. *WHO Guidelines on Hand Hygiene in Health Care: A Summary*. Geneva: WHO, 2009. Available from: https://apps.who.int/iris/handle/10665/70126

Laboratory Design, Equipment and Consumables for Oocyte Retrieval

Stephen Harbottle

9.1 Introduction

Since the inception of in vitro fertilisation (IVF) as a revolutionary and ground-breaking infertility treatment more than 40 years ago, we have witnessed huge scientific and research investment culminating in a plethora of procedural changes, technological advances, and service and legislative developments, which have served to increase the safety and efficacy of the treatment process worldwide. However, the biology and scientific principles that underpin the laboratory elements of IVF treatment remain the same, as does the vulnerability of human gametes and embryos to process-related stresses they would not normally be exposed to in vivo.

The oocyte is the largest human cell and is uniquely purposed for sexual reproduction. In terms of IVF, oocyte quality is one of the most significant determinant factors when prognosticating treatment outcome [1]. The human oocyte, despite its pivotal role in the continuation of the species, is inherently vulnerable to changes in temperature and pH and was never intended to spend a moment outside the body. For example, an apparently modest reduction in temperature from 37 to 35°C will result in depolymerisation of the meiotic spindle, which, although reversible, may result in subsequent aneuploidy [2] and certainly a reduction in treatment efficacy. It is well known and accepted that a successful culture system is a consistent culture system [Professor R. G. Edwards, conference communication].

IVF, by virtue of its very nature, necessitates the surgical harvesting, identification, processing and insemination of oocytes to occur outside the body. Intracytoplasmic sperm injection (ICSI) adds an additional layer of complexity to this process by expecting the oocyte to first tolerate the mechanical removal of the cumulus oophorus cells, which naturally surround it, and then respond, in a 'biologically appropriate' manner, to the intrusive mechanical injection of a sperm into its inner vestments, and fertilise. The oocyte must then go through multiple cellular divisions to form an embryo and ultimately a blastocyst capable of resulting in pregnancy and live birth following the final stage of the IVF process, embryo transfer.

For IVF success rates to be optimised, the oocytes must reach the entry point of the laboratory culture system in the best possible condition. The oocyte must be protected from unnecessary environmental and mechanical stresses at every point in the IVF or ICSI process, a journey that begins, in laboratory terms at least, with the oocyte retrieval procedure. Historically, oocyte retrieval procedures were performed laparoscopically. However, for the last 25 years, the preferred technique for routine surgical retrieval of oocytes has been transvaginal ultrasound-guided oocyte retrieval (TVOR).

TVOR is a process that spans two locations (oocyte retrieval room and laboratory) and two specialties (clinical and scientific), and the contribution of each is pivotal. It is important that the clinic recognises the importance of allowing these processes to synergise and not be regarded as discrete.

When harvested, oocytes are surrounded by a cellular mass comprising cumulus cells referred to as the cumulus–oocyte complex (COC). In this chapter, we consider the laboratory elements of TVOR and how these considerations play a pivotal role in ensuring that the harvested COCs are identified, processed and incubated in such a way as to optimise the oocyte condition for onward fertilisation and embryo development. These processes must compliment the efforts of the clinical team in the oocyte retrieval room, not conflict with them. To achieve this, careful consideration must be given to the key elements involved in the process, which are:

- Robust laboratory design
- Process and personnel flow

- Environmental considerations
- Equipment requirements
- Selection of appropriate consumables and reagents
- Monitoring of critical equipment
- Procedural considerations
- Operator training and competence
- Consistency, precision and accuracy.

Although often regarded as a simple procedure, the laboratory element of the TVOR procedure is a significant responsibility. The laboratory scientist involved not only has to ensure that each follicular aspirate is examined in a timely manner but also that every oocyte is identified, harvested and stored in a way that does not compromise its capacity to fertilise and subsequently form an embryo of the highest possible quality. The laboratory considerations required to succeed in this challenge will be considered in this chapter.

9.2 Laboratory Design

The journey of the oocyte from the follicle to the first IVF culture dish should be as short, efficient, controllable and traceable as possible. The oocyte retrieval room should be adjacent to the laboratory (Figure 9.1), and ideally the two should be directly connected by a transfer hatch to allow the laboratory scientist immediate access to the harvested follicular

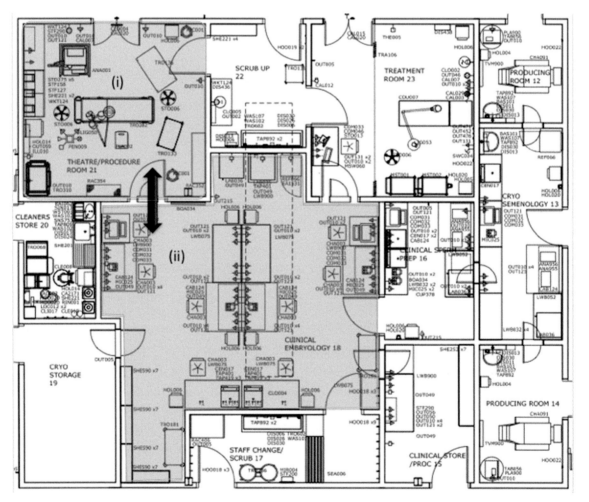

Figure 9.1 An architectural drawing of a well-designed assisted conception facility. Note how the oocyte retrieval room (i, shaded) and in vitro fertilisation laboratory (ii, shaded) are adjacent to one another and linked by a 'hatch in a door arrangement' (arrow) to allow efficient process flow and functional flexibility.

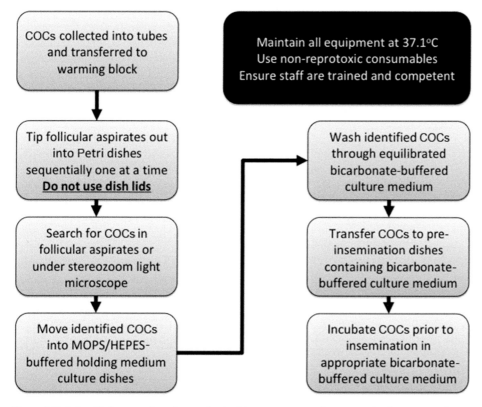

Figure 9.2 A simplified process flow diagram for the laboratory aspects of oocyte retrieval.

aspirates for identification and appropriate incubation of COCs. Ensuring that environmental stability is assured during the TVOR with regard to the procedural elements undertaken in both the oocyte retrieval room and the IVF laboratory is pivotal to the onward prognosis of treatment [1, 2].

9.2.1 Process and Personnel Flow

The laboratory elements of TVOR can be summarised very easily in a simple flow diagram (Figure 9.2). This does not, however, reflect the level of attention to detail, planning and validation required to ensure that the process is performed in a safe, efficient and biologically appropriate manner on every occasion.

Careful consideration must be given to the design and layout of the oocyte retrieval workspace within the laboratory. The TVOR process represents the oocyte entry point into the laboratory and the sequence of processes that follow it are of fundamental importance to the efficiency of the laboratory and the efficacy of the treatment services provided. The design of the space in which the science is performed

will dictate how people and processes flow, and should be carefully considered. For example, a door between two rooms allows personnel and processes to flow between the spaces. In a cleanroom laboratory environment, it is often the case that personnel flow needs to be restricted, yet processes must continue to flow. In such situations, 'transfer hatches' between spaces allow processes to flow 'through a wall'. In certain situations, it may be the case that a hybrid arrangement can be deployed where some functions of a space necessitate a door and others a hatch. The solution to this challenge is a hatch within a door arrangement (Figure 9.3), which ensures that spaces can be deployed to multiple purposes.

Another critical design element when considering laboratory processes is ensuring that the laboratory scientist can focus their complete attention on the procedure and that all of the consumables and equipment they require are close to hand. Ensuring that adequate staffing resources are available not just to perform the procedure but also to witness those procedures without staff having to move from one task to

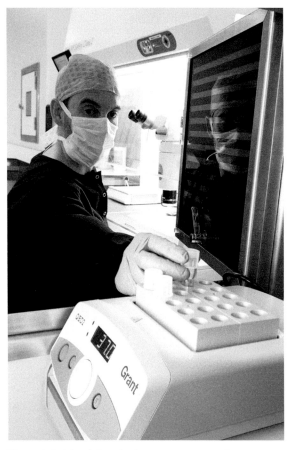

Figure 9.3 A 'hatch in a door' arrangement in use during transvaginal ultrasound-guided oocyte retrieval. Note that personnel flow between the two spaces is restricted to maintain laboratory containment, while follicular aspirates can freely move between the two spaces via the test-tube warmer to optimise procedural efficiency.

another is a key consideration in ensuring that the laboratory operates in a manner that is safe and compliant with the Human Fertilisation and Embryology Authority (HFEA) code of practice (CoP) [3]. Situations where operators need to cross paths should be avoided in a well-considered laboratory design, as it is such situations where the risk of procedural error or accident is at its most significant.

9.2.2 Environmental Considerations

The environment in which COCs are identified, washed and moved into culture forms an essential part of the IVF laboratory environment. The laboratory should maintain a positive-pressure cascade at all times. A positive-pressure cascade ensures that the

most critical area (the central IVF laboratory) is maintained at a higher pressure than the associate support rooms surrounding it (e.g. the oocyte retrieval room). By maintaining a pressure differential of approximately 15 Pa between rooms, it is possible to maintain high standards of cleanliness in the most critical areas of the facility, as any dust, dirt or potential pathogens are continually blown away from the highest pressure ('cleanest') room towards those at lower pressure or extract vents linked to the air handling unit delivering the pressure cascade.

Careful planning of these spaces and how they link together will not only allow the establishment of a robust and multilayered pressure cascade but also allow 30 or more complete air changes per hour within the laboratory space, to ensure that the air circulating in the laboratory does not itself prevent a risk to the culture system by accumulating toxins over time. The laboratory air itself should be passed through a recirculating filtration system containing activated carbon and HEPA filtration units and/or photocatalytic decontamination systems to ensure that pathogens such as microbes, volatile organic compounds and other chemically active compounds that may be detrimental to the culture system are continually removed.

Maintaining consistent environmental conditions within a range that does not cause stress to gametes and embryos is a key consideration in any effective laboratory design. The ambient levels of temperature, humidity and light intensity within the laboratory should be optimised and maintained, and measures taken to remove potentially harmful contaminants such as ultraviolet light from the laboratory using appropriate light tube filtration [4]. The same precautions should be adopted in the oocyte retrieval room to ensure that the COCs are not subject to any deleterious effects prior to entering the laboratory culture system.

9.3 Equipment Considerations

In the UK, the HFEA CoP defines the legal requirements and expected standards with regard to the equipment and materials used to perform all processes within a licensed fertility centre [3]. These statutory requirements are defined as a series of 'licence conditions' within the CoP and referenced by a 'T' number therein. In this chapter, we refer to these 'T' numbers to reference the relevant licence condition.

Laboratory equipment should be fit for purpose and appropriately installed, validated, maintained and operated in accordance with the manufacturer's specifications (T23 and T24 [3]). A list of the key equipment required to perform TVOR is provided below. This list is not exhaustive, and in some clinics, additional equipment may be required to adhere to local procedural requirements:

- Class II cabinet, 1,200 mm width, to allow adequate room around the microscope area for local incubation and ergonomic location of consumables
- Stereo zoom light microscope
- Heated microscope stage
- Mini bench-top incubator
- Test-tube warmer
- Manual or electronic witnessing system
- Laboratory chair with safety castors.

9.3.1 Optimising the Oocyte Retrieval Workstation

The oocyte retrieval workstation (Figure 9.4) should be located as close to the oocyte retrieval room as possible to ensure that test tubes containing follicular aspirates are not exposed to ambient temperatures outside any form of warming device for any longer than absolutely necessary. It should be clutter free, containing only the equipment and consumables necessary to perform one TVOR procedure, and should be thoroughly cleaned down with all consumables disposed of between every procedure.

All procedures involving the manipulation of gametes or embryos should be performed in a controlled environment with appropriate air quality. In the UK, this requirement is defined as a licence condition (T20 [3]) within the HFEA CoP as:

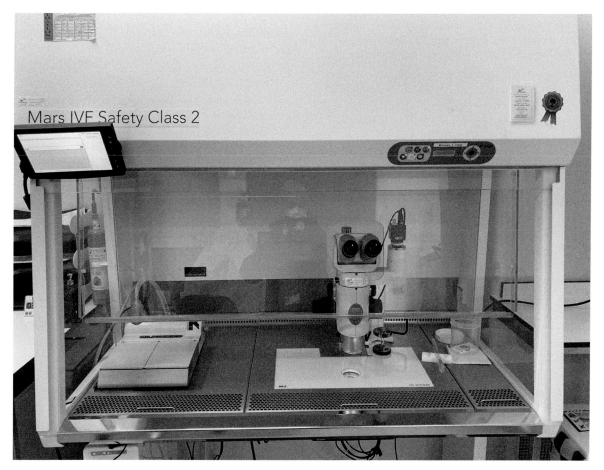

Figure 9.4 A typical in vitro fertilisation laboratory workstation arrangement to enable rapid and efficient transfer, and analysis of follicular aspirates while maintaining environmental stability during the procedure.

Table 9.1. Clean air device classification: maximum permitted number of particles per m³ equal to or greater than the tabulated size [5]

	At rest		In operation	
Grade	0.5 μm	5.0 μm	0.5 μm	5.0 μm
A	3,520	20	3,520	20
B	3,520	29	352,000	2,900
C	352,000	2,900	3,520,000	29,000
D	3,520,000	29,000	Not defined	Not defined

Table 9.2. Recommended limits for microbiological monitoring of clean areas during operation [5]

	Recommended limits for microbial contamination[a]			
Grade	Air sample (cfu/ m³)	Settle plates (diameter 90 mm) (cfu/4 hours)[b]	Contact plates (diameter 55 mm) (cfu/plate)	Glove print five fingers (cfu/ glove)
A	<1	<1	<1	<1
B	10	5	5	5
C	100	50	25	–
D	200	100	50	–

cfu, Colony-forming units.
[a] These are average values.
[b] Individual settle plates may be exposed for less than 4 hours.

In premises where the processing of gametes and embryos exposes them to the environment, the processing must take place in an environment of at least grade C air quality, with a background environment of at least grade D air quality as defined in the current European Guide to Good Manufacturing Practice (GMP_ Annex 1 and Directive 2003/94/EC). It must be demonstrated and documented that the chosen environment achieves the quality and safety required.

This legislative requirement is intended to ensure that, in the context of the TVOR process, the COCs are harvested in an environment where the air quality is such that it does not cause harm to the oocytes or put the culture system at risk of contamination. The grade of air is verified by a combination of air sampling using a portable particle counter to determine atmospheric particulate levels (Table 9.1) and settle and/or contact plates to determine levels of microbial contamination (Table 9.2) [5]. A schedule should be established as part of the laboratory verification plan to ensure that air quality is determined at regular intervals. As confidence in the facility and verification schedule increases over time, the frequency of air-quality sampling assessments may decrease but should never be less than 6-monthly. Where laboratory air quality falls below the designated standard, a reactive cleaning plan should be implemented. Regular 6-monthly deep cleaning of the laboratory and associated support rooms is recommended using appropriate gamete- and embryo-friendly cleaning solutions and/or vaporised hydrogen peroxide gas sterilisation at a time when there is no clinical activity ongoing in the laboratory.

It is not just the air quality that should be regarded as a key-determining factor in reducing the risk of harm to COCs; the efficiency with which the laboratory scientist can work should also be carefully and thoroughly considered:

- The laboratory scientist should be able to pick up COC tubes directly from the test-tube warmer without a need to move from the workstation.
- The workstation should be configured in such a way as to ensure that it is clutter free and all equipment is readily accessible.
- The layout should ensure that risk of avoidable stress and loss or damage to COCs is minimised.
- The workstation should be designed and configured so that it provides an ergonomic workspace for both left- and right-handed laboratory scientists.
- The TVOR procedure represents an entry point into the laboratory culture system. As such, appropriate manual or electronic witnessing procedures should be in place to ensure an effective chain of custody is in place from the moment the COCs enter the culture system (section 18.4(a) in [3]).

9.3.2 Monitoring and Maintenance of Critical Equipment

Validation and verification of procedures forms an integral part of the laboratory quality management system (T72 [3]). In the context of the TVOR process, all equipment that is deployed to maintain environmental conditions during the procedure should be regularly, and ideally continually, monitored to ensure that it is operating within the parameters specified in the associated protocol and any functional specification documentation. It is critical to ensure that independent monitoring of all such parameters is performed to ensure that, should any equipment fault develop that causes a shift in set point and/or failure of the built-in monitoring probe, this is immediately detected and an alarm triggered so that corrective actions can be taken to reduce the impact of any resultant harm. Examples of equipment assessments that should be subject to such independent monitoring, validation and verification include:

- Test-tube warmer temperature assessment
- Heated-stage temperature assessment
- Consumable items via batch-specific toxicity testing
- Incubator temperature, CO_2 and O_2 concentration, and humidity.

These validation and verification processes should be extended to consider the necessary consumables and culture medium deployed, as well as operator competence, as follows [6]:

- Culture medium temperature and pH
- Procedural efficacy
- Operator competence via establishment and monitoring of appropriate key performance indicators.

In addition to robust equipment monitoring, it is also of critical importance to ensure that all equipment is maintained and serviced in accordance with the specifications of the manufacturer (T26 [3]). Laboratory managers should also risk assess processes and procedures to ensure that adequate, well-maintained equipment is available to provide adequate redundancy. This process includes ensuring that the facility holds more than one piece of equipment that is deemed to be essential to a process. In terms of TVOR from the laboratory aspect, this may include, but is not limited to:

- Class II biological safety cabinet
- Stereo zoom microscope
- Test-tube warmer.

Where procedures cannot be completed safely without specific pieces of equipment, consideration must be made to ensuring that the centre's equipment inventory contains more than one similar piece of equipment, even if that equipment is repurposed rather than lying dormant, as long as it is appropriately serviced and maintained and readily available in case an equipment failure should occur. These considerations are more pressing in smaller units where the caseload itself does not lend itself to a need, based on activity levels, for equipment to be duplicated for the purposes of routine service delivery.

Where such redundancy cannot be resourced, a risk assessment should be performed and a robust arrangement put in place with another licensed fertility centre to ensure that patient care can be transferred seamlessly and without delay to ensure that treatment processes are not compromised any more than absolutely necessary due to equipment failure.

9.4 Consumable and Reagent Requirements for TVOR

Laboratory consumables should be selected on their quality and appropriateness (Figure 9.5). Where available, consumables CE marked as medical devices should be preferentially used (T30 [3]). Careful selection of consumables should also be made based on laboratory preference, cost appraisal, supply-chain efficiency and an awareness of the risk of reprotoxicity [7]. Appropriate toxicity testing should be performed by the manufacturer at source via a mouse embryo assay and may be repeated on site by the clinic using sperm toxicity testing. It should be noted that a high degree of heterogeneity exists with regard to the reprotoxicity tests performed by manufacturers when validating their IVF disposable devices and that currently no regulations exist on this issue [8].

Where mouse embryo assay-tested consumables are not available, in-house toxicity testing should be performed on every individual batch of consumables deployed. Do not assume that consumables cannot be reprotoxic; 13 out of 36 consumable products commonly used in the IVF laboratory were found to be toxic to gametes and embryos [7]. These products included surgical gloves, oocyte collection needle tubing, TVOR needles, sterile Pasteur pipettes and one type of IVF Petri dish [7]. The lids of Petri dishes should not be used to tip out follicular aspirates for COC identification, as the CE mark applied to the dish does not cover the use of the lid for that purpose.

An example of a list of laboratory consumables for TVOR is provided below:

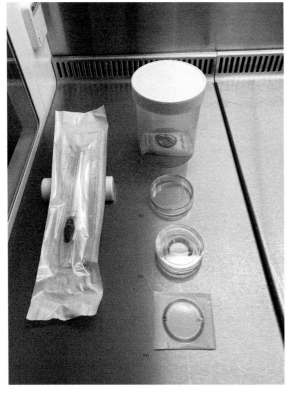

Figure 9.5 The consumables required to perform oocyte retrieval. (i) Follicular aspirate discard pot with a superabsorbent liquid-absorbing sachet. (ii) 60 mm CE-marked sterile Petri dish (do not use lids!) (iii) Equilibrated dish containing MOPS- or HEPES-buffered in vitro fertilisation culture medium overlaid with mineral oil. (iv) Radio frequency identification dish label for use with electronic witnessing system. (v) COC aspiration pipette (600 μm).

- COC aspiration pipette (glass or plastic ≥600 μm diameter).
- 15 ml test tubes to harvest follicular aspirates.
- 60 or 90 mm Petri dishes for tipping out follicular aspirates for the identification of COCs.
- Discard pot containing a superabsorbent liquid-absorbing sachet for disposal of follicular aspirates after screening for the presence of COCs.
- MOPS (3-(N-morpholino)propanesulfonic acid)- or HEPES (4-(2-hydroxyethyl)-1-piperazineethanesulfonic acid)-buffered IVF culture medium for identification and short-term storage of COCs ('holding dishes').
- Bicarbonate-buffered IVF culture medium for COC washing and equilibration of COCs ('wash dishes').
- Bicarbonate-buffered IVF culture medium for COC incubation post-washing prior to insemination ('storage dishes').

- IVF-quality mineral oil for overlaying holding, wash and storage dishes.
- Appropriate personal protective equipment (PPE; non-latex laboratory gloves, surgical mask and surgical hat).
- Dish labels containing three unique identifiers (name, date of birth and clinic number).
- Electronic witnessing system labels (radio frequency identification or barcode reading systems).

Culture medium choice should be based on preferred supplier of a CE-marked and validated IVF culture medium. Culture systems should be designed to minimise gamete stress during procedures outside a controlled incubator environment and thoroughly validated for this purpose. It is important to be aware that oocytes lack robust mechanisms to regulate their internal pH, so a strategy must be developed, validated and implemented to maintain an optimal pH during COC retrieval procedures [9]. CE-marked and validated MOPS- or HEPES-buffered culture medium designed to support oocytes outside the incubator for protracted periods of time are readily commercially available from a number of reputable suppliers and should be considered for the purpose of COC retrieval. Bicarbonate-buffered culture medium designed for the culture of gametes and embryos within a stable incubator environment with an enriched atmospheric concentration of CO_2 (usually 5–6%) should not be used for any procedure where the gametes or embryos will be outside the incubator for more than 180 seconds, as control of pH and temperature will be lost after this time (Cambridge IVF, UK, unpublished validation data). The use of a local mini-incubator at the point of procedure within the oocyte retrieval class II biological safety cabinet is recommended to prevent oocyte cooling during the TVOR procedure and the resultant damage this can lead to [2].

All consumables must be batch controlled, and clinics should deploy a traceability system to ensure that, for every TVOR performed, comprehensive records are available not only with regard to the personnel involved in the procedure but also the exact lot numbers of all consumables and culture media deployed (T99 [3]).

9.5 Identification of COCs in the Laboratory

The oocyte retrieval as a process has been described in Chapter 5; however a synopsis of the process is relevant to this chapter. Oocytes are most commonly collected by TVOR using a specific oocyte collection needle connected via a foot-actuated suction pump to a test tube into which the follicular aspirate is harvested. The process may or may not involve the flushing of ovarian follicles with appropriate culture medium.

The journey of the oocyte begins with its aspiration from the follicle via the TVOR needle and onwards into fine-bore sterile silicone tubing of approximately 1 m in length until it is collected in a sterile 15ml test tube in a test-tube warmer, which is accessible by the laboratory scientist directly from their workstation. Follicular aspirates are then sequentially analysed for the presence or absence of COCs under the microscope.

COCs are visible to the (trained) human eye and readily identifiable using a microscope at a relatively low level of magnification ($\times 10$–20 range). It is common practice for more than one follicle to be drained per test tube received, so it is important that communication between the practitioner performing the TVOR and the scientist in the laboratory is effective to maximise COC yield.

9.6 Procedural Precision and Accuracy

Best practice in the IVF laboratory is based on two key principles: working with precision and working with accuracy. It is the duty of a competent laboratory scientist to ensure that every patient is provided with a consistently high standard of care from the moment their gametes enter the laboratory until the end point of their treatment cycle. Systems should be designed and staff trained and competency assessed regularly to ensure that validated procedures are followed, intra-operator variation is minimised and equipment is maintained. These measures are intended to ensure that the laboratory scientist, the equipment and consumables, and the TVOR process itself do not contribute any detrimental factor. To this end, the laboratory scientist must adopt and maintain meticulous and consistent attention to detail, awareness of process flow and certain levels of skill (Figure 9.6).

The equipment, consumable and procedural choices made by the clinic play a pivotal part in this process, and where procedural changes are proposed, an impact assessment must be performed to ensure that they do not add any risk or complexity that may have a detrimental effect on the process and the subsequent treatment outcome.

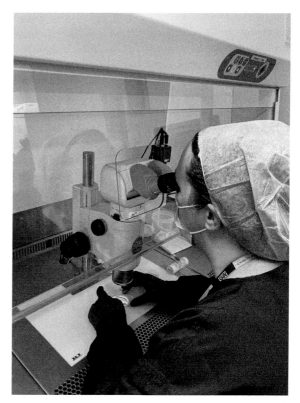

Figure 9.6 A clinical embryologist performing an oocyte retrieval procedure wearing appropriate personal protective equipment to perform the task safely and protect both themselves and the cumulus–oocyte complexes collected. Note that the workstation is well organised and clutter free, containing only the equipment and consumables required for the one procedure undertaken at any one time.

9.7 Additional Equipment and Procedural Considerations

In this chapter, we have considered and defined the key elements involved in the laboratory aspects of TVOR with regard to facilities, equipment, consumables and processes for a 'typical' fertility clinic. We should, however, conclude by briefly considering other less common considerations, which may not be relevant to all clinics but may influence the manner in which TVOR should be performed.

9.7.1 Considerations for TVOR for Virus-Positive Patients

It is not uncommon for fertility centres to offer fertility treatment to people who have tested positive for conditions such as human immunodeficiency virus

73

(HIV) infection or hepatitis B or C. Such cases are commonly referred to as 'high risk'. In such circumstances, additional precautions should be taken to ensure that the risk of contamination or transmission of the virus is minimised. Centres should develop a strategy to manage high-risk cases in a way that protects the patient, the staff members, other patients and the laboratory culture system from inadvertent virus inoculation. The following additional measures should be considered:

- Virus-positive patients should be last on the oocyte retrieval list.
- A spill kit should be readily available in case of accidental spillage of potentially virus-positive biological fluids or contaminated materials during the procedure.
- All non-essential equipment and consumables should be removed from the workstation prior to the procedure.
- The class II safety cabinet used during the procedure should be allowed to run on high flow for 30 minutes following decontamination to allow adequate air changes before it is used for any other laboratory process or purpose.
- All equipment used during the TVOR procedure should be decontaminated with an appropriate antiviral solution validated to be effective against the relevant virus, and equipment should not be used again until it has been cleaned in accordance with the manufacturer's instructions.
- Additional PPE should be deployed including an overgown, eye protection and double-layer gloving.
- Where possible, a second member of the laboratory team should act as an assistant during the procedure to avoid the high-risk operator needing to move from their workstation for any reason.

9.7.2 Considerations for Offsite Oocyte Retrieval under a Transport IVF Arrangement

Although it is less common than it once was, some centres still operate a transport IVF arrangement. This should not be confused with a satellite IVF service. In transport IVF arrangements, COCs are harvested at one location, usually without a dedicated specialist IVF laboratory, and transferred in a transport incubator to the central laboratory for onward

processing, insemination and completion of fertility treatment.

In such circumstances, careful thought must be given not only to ensure that staff working at the transport service are trained and competent to perform their roles but also that all of the equipment and consumables used to harvest COCS are validated and subject to appropriate traceability controls. In addition, careful consideration must be given to the mechanistic and procedural elements of the transportation process to ensure that the quality of the oocytes is not compromised during transport to the main laboratory.

9.8 Summary

To ensure each treatment cycle is given the best possible chance of a positive outcome requires harvesting and preparation of gametes of the highest possible quality. TVOR is invasive, unnatural, and places significant and unavoidable stresses on the oocytes. These stresses, if not well managed, may reduce the viability and potential of the oocytes harvested. By developing an awareness of the importance of optimal laboratory process flow and making wise choices with regard to equipment and consumables, we can be successful in optimising the environment in which TVOR is performed from both a clinical and laboratory perspective. In addition, we have an absolute duty to our patients to ensure that, as competent and dedicated laboratory scientists, we are working with an absolute commitment to precision and accuracy during every procedure we perform.

Only by doing so are we able to ensure that treatment cycles start out on the best possible footing to thrive, form viable pregnancies, and ultimately deliver a safe and healthy singleton live birth as often as possible.

9.9 Final Thoughts: COVID-19

In early 2020, the way we live our lives was changed in a way that was unprecedented in our lifetimes. For the first time in its history, the HFEA issued legislation that temporarily suspended the treatment licences of every licensed fertility clinic in the UK (GD0014 [3]). In order to resume provision of fertility treatment services, licensed centres were obligated to not only review protocols and processes but also risk assess patient and staff flow within the centre, the availability of appropriate PPE and assure themselves that their supply chain would not be subject to volatility, which could compromise patient care.

The true fallout of the COVID-19 pandemic is not yet fully understood at the time of writing; however, it is clear that the way we approach the delivery of medical treatment services has changed, and centres are encouraged to continue to review their practices to ensure that patient and staff safety is protected by adhering to protocols that are intended to reduce the risks associated with viral pathogens. For example, oocyte retrieval lists may need to be shorter with longer gaps between cases to allow for additional COVID-19-related precautions such as dedicated donning and doffing areas, additional cleaning and sterilisation measures, allowing more air changes, and considering necessary social distancing recommendations in the way both patients and staff flow through the building.

The intended outcome is, of course, the same but the optimal methodology to achieve this objective has changed significantly and most probably will remain so for the foreseeable future.

References

1. Nelson SM, Lawlor DA. Predicting live birth, preterm delivery, and low birth weight in infants born from in vitro fertilisation: a prospective study of 144,018 treatment cycles. *PLoS Med* 2011;**8**(1):e1000386. doi: 10.1371/journal.pmed.1000386.

2. Pickering SJ, Braude PR, Johnson MH, Cant A, Currie J. Transient cooling to room temperature can cause irreversible disruption of the meiotic spindle in the human oocyte. *Fertil Steril* 1990;**54**(1):102–8. doi: 10.1016/s0015-0282(16)53644-9

3. Human Fertilisation and Embryology Authority (HEFA). *Code of Practice*, 9th ed. London: HEFA, 2018. Available from: https://portal.hfea.gov.uk/knowledge-base/read-the-code-of-practice/

4. Cairo Consensus Group. 'There is only one thing that is truly important in an IVF laboratory: everything.' Cairo Consensus Guidelines on IVF Culture Conditions. *Reprod Biomed Online* 2020;**40**(1):33–60. doi: 10.1016/j.rbmo.2019.10.003

5. European Commission. *The Rules Governing Medicinal Products in the European Union, Volume 4. EU Guidelines to Good Manufacturing Practice Medicinal Products for Human and Veterinary Use. Annex 1. Manufacture of Sterile Medicinal Products.* Brussels: European Commission, 2008. https://ec.europa.eu/health/sites/health/files/files/eudralex/vol-4/2008_11_25_gmp-an1_en.pdf

6. ESHRE Special Interest Group of Embryology and Alpha Scientists in Reproductive Medicine. The Vienna consensus: report of an expert meeting on the development of ART laboratory performance indicators. *Reprod Biomed Online* 2017;**35**(5):494–510. doi: 10.1016/j.rbmo.2017.06.015

7. Nijs M, Franssen K, Cox A, et al. Reprotoxicity of intrauterine insemination and in vitro fertilization–embryo transfer disposables and products: a 4-year survey. *Fertil Steril* 2008;**92**(2):527–35. doi: 10.1016/j.fertnstert.2008.07.011

8. Delaroche L, Oger P, Genauzeau E, et al. Embryotoxicity testing of IVF disposables: how do manufacturers test? *Hum Reprod* 2020;**35**(2):283–92.

9. Swain J. Optimizing the culture environment in the IVF laboratory: impact of pH and buffer capacity on gamete and embryo quality. *Reprod Biomed Online* 2010;**21**(1):6–16. doi: 10.1016/j.rbmo.2010.03.012

Quality Management Requirements for Oocyte Collection

Lucy Wood and Rachel Cutting

10.1 Quality Management in the IVF Unit

A robust quality management system (QMS) in an in vitro fertilisation (IVF) unit is imperative to its success and ongoing improvement. The purpose of the QMS is to ensure that every aspect of the running of the unit, from laboratory procedures to patient satisfaction, is monitored and optimised. Put simply, the QMS is essential for good practice. It is, or should be, the backbone of the service. An effective QMS will use risk-based thinking in a process approach to avoid deviations from the clinic's planned objectives. This chapter will consider how quality management can be successfully implemented during the oocyte collection procedure.

Although not a regulatory requirement in every country, implementing a QMS is stipulated in licence condition T32 from the Human Fertilisation and Embryo Authority (HFEA) in the UK and laboratory guidelines from the European Society of Human Reproduction and Embryology (ESHRE) [1]. The HFEA states that: 'The centre must put in place a quality management system and implement this system to continually improve the quality and effectiveness of the service provided in accordance with the conditions of this licence and the guidance on good practice as set out in the HFEA's Code of Practice' [2]. Effective quality management provides evidence to our regulators that we are consistently working within the requirements of the law.

Further to regulatory requirements, the QMS itself can be certified against criteria set by the International Organisation for Standardisation (ISO) [3]. ISO are responsible for publishing standards that can be implemented across a multitude of sectors and industries; ISO 9001:2015 is based on quality management principals and acts to assist organisations in perfecting their QMS. In order to gain certification,

the clinic must demonstrate through official inspection of documented records that their QMS meets the exacting criteria set out in the standard. This certification is recognised internationally as a stamp of approval that the receiving organisation is dedicated to continual improvement and customer satisfaction. Although not compulsory, compliance with ISO 9001:2015 will satisfy HFEA's requirements.

To fully grasp the topic of quality management, it is helpful to understand the terminology that comes with it. Quality management comprises quality control, quality assurance and quality improvement, each with its own unique definition but all contributing to the same goal [4]. Quality control involves specifying limits for the measurable aspects of a process, monitoring them regularly and taking any necessary remedial action to stay within these limits, for example, setting an acceptable temperature range for the fluid within the egg collection tube while in the electronic tube warmer (Figure 10.1A). Quality assurance is the collective term for all quality activities that are carried out to ensure that the service is sufficiently fit for purpose, which includes quality control. Activities such as audits, training and process validation all contribute to quality assurance for egg collection. Quality improvement concentrates on producing better outcomes with greater efficiency. Improvements can vary in scale; implementing multiple small quality improvements, or 'marginal gains', can lead to a notable improvement in pregnancy rate. For example, an extra oocyte rinse to remove handling medium and blood cells is a small addition that could provide a slightly healthier and more appropriate environment for the incubated oocyte (Figure 10.1B). Larger-scale improvements are usually the result of periodic scientific breakthroughs, such as switching to a low-O_2 culture system to closer mimic the oviduct [5]. In both instances, the alteration must be fully validated before change can take place and

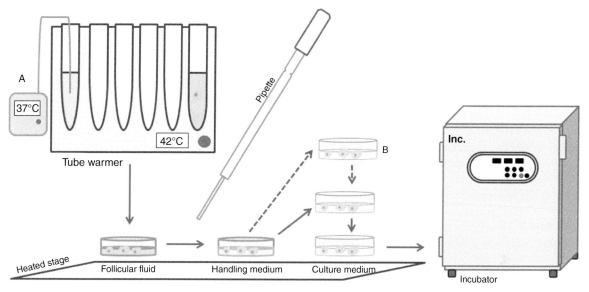

A

37°C

Tube warmer

42°C

Pipette

B

Inc.

Heated stage

Follicular fluid

Handling medium

Culture medium

Incubator

Figure 10.1 The laboratory processing of oocytes during egg collection. (A) External thermometer probe for validating tube warmer temperature setting. (B) Inclusion of an extra wash step in culture medium. A black and white version of this figure will appear in some formats. For the colour version, refer to the plate section.

subsequently monitored to ensure that it is not detrimental to the process. Assessing the fertilisation rate before and after any 'improvements' can help decipher their effectiveness.

10.2 Top-Quality Egg Collections

Quality management is multifaceted. It runs deep through the laboratory process and infiltrates every imaginable aspect of egg collection. From choosing equipment to training staff, checking the temperature of the workstation or designing paperwork, quality management is there.

In the laboratory, quality management ensures that each element of the egg collection process is optimised to protect the egg during transit from the ovary to the incubator (Figure 10.1). Potential physical risks to the egg such as temperature fluctuations, physical damage and infectious agents are carefully controlled to ensure each oocyte makes a safe journey into culture. Components such as equipment, consumables and choice of medium should be selected and validated prior to their implementation to ensure they are fit for purpose. The laboratory conditions and operator competence are also major considerations when optimising egg collection, and close monitoring of the entire process is critical for success;

a fault in any aspect of the procedure could lead to catastrophe.

10.2.1 Temperature Control and Equipment Validation

Maintaining oocyte temperature at 37°C throughout the egg collection procedure is critical; allowing the oocyte to cool to room temperature risks disruption of the meiotic spindle, a structure essential for producing euploid embryos [6]. All equipment used to maintain temperature during the egg collection procedure must be validated to ensure it is fit for this purpose. The heated stage, for example, has the purpose of maintaining the handling medium within the Petri dish at 37°C. Upon installing the heated stage, an installation and operational qualification should be undertaken to provide documented evidence that it is fit for purpose by performing a series of specific tests. The tests would include confirmation that supporting documents (e.g. instruction manuals) are present, all components of the heated stage (e.g. temperature settings) are in full working order and temperature mapping has established the temperature distribution under normal working conditions. All temperature measurements should be taken using the readings displayed on the equipment alongside an external calibrated probe as assurance that the displayed reading is accurate. A certificate of calibration for the external temperature probe will also need to be provided as well as considerations for the uncertainty of the measurement.

The temperature of the stage is not necessarily indicative of the temperature the oocyte will be held at; this can only be ascertained by creating an exact replica of the egg collection dish and measuring the temperature of the medium within it. If the type of dish used is substituted for another, a revalidation must take place due to variations in design. Some dishes will sit flush to the heated stage while others may have a small gap of a few millimetres. This differing proximity of the culture well to the heated stage will affect the temperature of the media and invalidate the previous temperature settings. It should be considered that the temperature of the heated stage can be affected by the bulb used for the inbuilt microscope, and the temperature may fluctuate across the area of the stage. When taking measurements for validation purposes, the bulb must be switched on just as it would be during egg collection. The heat from the bulb may increase the temperature of the medium and should be assessed to ensure it will not have a damaging effect. The whole of the stage should be validated for reassurance that the eggs will be at the correct temperature regardless of their positioning; any areas of the heated stage that fall out of range should be marked for avoidance.

The tube warmer is used to help maintain the temperature of the aspirated follicular fluid prior to the egg search. The temperature of the oocyte environment within the tube will depend almost exclusively on the tube warmer temperature setting; therefore, it is paramount that this setting is correct. Due to inevitable heat loss from tube warmer to the tube and to the fluid within, this setting will be an overestimate and will not accurately reflect the temperature of the oocyte environment. To ascertain the temperature of the fluid, an external calibrated thermometer probe can be inserted into a mock fluid-filled test tube held within the warmer (Figure 10.1A), and the temperature setting adjusted on the tube warmer until the desired fluid temperature of 37°C is reached.

This equipment validation process should be repeated regularly (at least every 2 years) through an equipment qualification review (EQR) to demonstrate ongoing validation. An EQR is also required following an equipment repair to ensure it has been carried out to a sufficient standard. The EQR will assess that servicing contracts for maintenance of the equipment are in place via a third party and are regularly updated. Equipment involved during the egg collection process that requires validation includes the oocyte collection pump, flow hood, heated stages, incubators and test-tube warmers.

10.2.2 Equipment, Media and Consumable Selection

Quality management includes the selection of fit-for-purpose equipment, media and consumables that will work harmoniously together to provide a stable environment for the collected egg. Optimising the system will take careful consideration and should factor in the size and workload of the laboratory, the manufacturers' recommendations and any cost implications. If we take the example of selecting which incubator to install, we have various factors to consider. Size, shape, inclusion of individual compartments and the speed of temperature recovery or gas stabilisation should all be deliberated prior to purchase, as well as additional functions such as inclusion of time-lapse technology [7]. We need to be assured that the CO_2 levels within the incubator can maintain our chosen oocyte culture medium at a suitable pH level during routine workload. In-house validation (which can be troublesome and/or expensive) or choosing to follow the manufacturers' recommendations are both ways of achieving the necessary assurance [8]. It may be advantageous to use media from the same manufacturer for both handling (outside the incubator) and culture (inside the incubator) of oocytes; however, you might find using a combination of suppliers works best for your culture system. Media, consumable and equipment options are plentiful and there will be multiple 'right choices'. An effective QMS will help you find the right combination of products for optimum results in your own laboratory through validation, frequent monitoring of results and reporting any undesirable observations that could potentially be attributed to your choices.

10.2.3 Laboratory Conditions

For egg collection to be successful, the laboratory environment must be suitably clean. The presence of microbes (bacteria, viruses and fungi) or air-polluting volatile organic compounds (VOCs) within the laboratory is detrimental to embryo development and patient safety. In the UK, laboratory air quality must comply with the stipulations of HFEA of at least a grade D background air environment; this tightens to a grade C environment for gamete and embryo processing [2]. Definitions of air-quality grades are defined in the current European Guide to Good Manufacturing Practice [9]. High-efficiency particulate air or HEPA filters can minimise unwanted particle levels within the laboratory and have been shown to positively affect IVF outcomes; however, unwanted particles can be present within the air, on surfaces, inside the incubator or on laboratory personnel [10]. These minute threats are largely undetectable by the embryologist and should be tested for frequently with particle counts and microbiology testing as part of laboratory quality control. Elevated levels could contribute to a reduced live birth rate and must be investigated.

VOCs are a specific family of toxic substances that are able to dissolve into culture media or oil and interfere with oocyte biochemistry. The two most common VOCs found in IVF laboratories are ethanol and isopropyl alcohol, which are metabolised into acetaldehyde and formaldehyde, respectively. These compounds are known carcinogens and mutagens and, unsurprisingly, have been shown to have majorly deleterious effects on embryo development [11]. These biologically damaging chemicals can arise from a variety of sources such as laboratory furniture, incubator components, plasticware, HVAC (heating, ventilation and air conditioning) air intake, cleaning products and laboratory staff. In some cases, levels can be reduced by allowing sufficient time for 'off-gassing' of new equipment and consumables in a suitably clean environment away from the gamete-handling laboratory. The laboratory environment can be improved by installing carbon filters that adsorb unwanted airborne chemicals, and using inline gas filters to purify the gases used for embryo culture is also likely to be of benefit [12]. Expert consensus points on air quality have been reached and published to guide management of VOCs in the IVF laboratory [11].

10.2.4 Reprotoxicity

The oocyte encounters numerous instruments and solutions, which all have their effects on viability and ultimately the success of the procedure. As per the HFEA guidelines, all consumables and media that come into contact with the oocyte must be tested for toxicity and be fully traceable through batch control [2]. In order to establish the functionality and toxicity of each batch, a mouse embryo assay can be performed and results reported through a certificate of analysis accompanying each delivery from an accredited supplier. It is important that the batch number of any consumable that the egg will encounter is recorded and can readily be accessed, allowing no uncertainty as to which batch was in use. In the event of a faulty batch being reported, eggs that have been in contact with the offending item can be identified quickly and accurately. Batch tracing can also be used for troubleshooting purposes. For example, we can eliminate any involvement of the plasticware when investigating an adverse outcome if the same batch has performed to standard elsewhere.

10.2.5 Risk Assessment

Risk-based thinking ensures a 'prophylactic management' ethos, i.e. prevention is better than cure, a method that has been implemented successfully to improve IVF quality management [4]. By being proactive and exploring the worst-case scenarios of what could and might happen, mistakes can be prevented. For example, if an IVF clinic choses to replace their current egg collection dish with a different product, the new item must be validated and risk assessed prior to its implementation, particularly if the product is not CE marked. The risk of using a non-CE-marked product must be quantified and weighed up against the drawbacks of keeping the original dish. For products that are not tested by mouse embryo assay as standard by the supplier (and therefore not CE marked for IVF), a sperm survival assay can be performed as part of an in-house risk assessment [13]. Reprotoxicity testing will help quantify the risk, and dishes could be tested in tandem to assess their relative performance. Documenting the risk assessment of using a non-CE-marked product demonstrates that careful consideration has gone into the use of the product and may help avoid a 'non-conformance' during an inspection. This should only be the case if no other CE-marked product is available or it is deemed to pose a considerably greater risk to the oocyte.

Performing a risk assessment involves scoring the likelihood of an adverse event occurring against the

Likelihood	Consequence				
	Insignificant (1)	Minor (2)	Moderate (3)	Major (4)	Catastrophic (5)
Rare (1)	1	2	3	4	5
Unlikely (2)	2	4	6	8	10
Possible (3)	3	6	9	12	15
Likely (4)	4	8	12	16	20
Almost certain (5)	5	10	15	20	25

Figure 10.2 Risk rating during a risk assessment. A black and white version of this figure will appear in some formats. For the colour version, refer to the plate section.

severity of the negative consequences. Both are scored from 1 to 5, with 1 being the least likely to occur or causing minimal disruption and 5 being almost certain to occur or having a catastrophic impact (Figure 10.2). The scores are multiplied together to give a risk rating from low (3 or below) to extreme (15 or above), which should be acted on accordingly. Actions can be taken to reduce the risk rating to a more acceptable level or eliminate the risk completely.

10.2.6 Traceability and Witnessing

During egg collection, there must be a robust system in place to unambiguous identify the owner of the gametes. The dish should be labelled with three separate patient identifiers such as name, date of birth and hospital number. The label should be legible and unobstructed to avoid it being misread during a witnessing step. At egg collection, the patient confirms their identity, which is checked against the dish labels through double witnessing, where two humans check the identifiers prior to dish use. This is documented by a physical signature on the paperwork. Electronic witnessing (such as RI Witness™) provides reassurance to all parties through an radio frequency identification (RFID)-tagged checking system that logs each movement of gametes or embryos, recording the exact date and time, and functioning as an alert system should the incorrect material be brought into the working area [14]. The record of events is stored on computer software ready to be analysed if needed. Each operator has their own login, and the system is able to incorporate the need for a second human

witness at crucial steps such as IVF insemination. Other electronic witnessing systems are available.

10.2.7 Supplier Accreditation

To confidently say that the egg collection procedure is as optimal as possible, all suppliers of services or manufacturers of goods associated with the egg collection must also be assessed for suitability. Suppliers can prove this by providing a certificate of accreditation as reassurance that they too adhere to a robust QMS, such as being ISO compliant [3]. Being able to demonstrate that all acquired laboratory products are subject to strict quality control helps eliminate the likelihood of their involvement in an undesirable outcome. Third-party agreements should be put in place between the accredited supplier and the clinic that specify the expectations of each party. For example, during egg collection, the heated stage is heavily relied upon and at regular intervals should be serviced and calibrated by the supplier to ensure it is continuing to perform adequately. Post-servicing, a certificate will be issued that confirms the temperature settings have been tested and recalibrated according to manufacturing standards (e.g. 37°C) and that the equipment used to perform the calibration has itself been calibrated to national standards. Following this, the clinic may need to adjust the temperature as per their own validation protocol as described previously. The third-party agreement with the supplier would state how often the product will be serviced and against which standards, the agreed price including any additional purchases that may be required for its function, the duration of the agreement and the responsibilities of either party. It would be unwise to assume that all suppliers of IVF products will provide a service that is up to scratch, and therefore the third-party agreement offers peace of mind from a quality management perspective and documents exactly what is required from either party, leaving no uncertainty. The contract protects the clinic from unexpected price increases, delays or shoddy workmanship. The agreed terms must be documented and a formal contract signed by both parties; it is not acceptable to omit this document because of a friendly or long-standing relationship with the supplier [4].

10.2.8 Operator Training and Competence

Adequate operator training and competence is essential for a successful egg collection. Competence can be measured by supervision of the trainee by a more senior embryologist who may check dishes for missed eggs. It will be set in the training policy how competency is assessed and a supervisor will sign off the trainee as 'competent' based on their speed, accuracy and confidence throughout the task. The assessment criteria should include the trainee's ability to work at pace and keep up with the clinical operator to avoid a backlog of tubes within the warming rack waiting for the egg search. If there is a high proportion of blood within these waiting tubes, clotting of the follicular fluid can occur leading to loss of gametes. Working within earshot of an experienced embryologist can offer valuable support for newly trained embryologists and reduce the occurrence of avoidable incidents during the nerve-wracking first procedures flying solo. The competence of every embryologist should be reassessed at least annually to reassure that the optimal protocol is consistently adhered to. Deviations from the protocol will be identified during this assessment, highlighting areas where retraining is required or potential updates to the protocol are necessary.

10.2.9 Documentation

Controlled documentation is crucially important for a successful QMS due to the strong emphasis on compliance and traceability within the IVF sector. Each current document should be approved, accessible and distinguishable with an identifying issue number; outdated versions should be archived and any unapproved versions removed. Documents can be managed using basic IT programmes (e.g. spreadsheets with hyperlinks to word-processed files) or by utilising quality management software (e.g. Q-pulse®). Documents relating to the oocyte retrieval include a standard operating procedure (SOP), a laboratory form to record the outcome and a standardised consent form to be signed prior to the procedure by the patient. Patient information leaflets and letter templates should also be controlled to ensure that patients do not receive inaccurate information, and that information is delivered in a standardised and approved way. A printed document displaying typos or out-of-date information suggests poor attention to detail and may damage the reputation of the clinic;. Document control will help to avoid this.

The SOP details which equipment should be used and instructs the embryologist how to carry out the egg collection procedure. The desired outcome should be clear, and all reagents necessary for the procedure should be listed. In addition, a good SOP should provide a source of reference for embryologists to explain not just how the procedure should be performed but also why it must be carried out that way. The SOP should be updated to reflect any protocol changes and reviewed at least annually via process validation to consider new research, techniques or products for implementation. The updated issue should be circulated to all laboratory staff members and the previous issue removed and archived. By adhering to the SOP, consistency between operators is promoted, which eliminates 'procedural differences' as a predictor of outcome. Any 'short cuts' implemented by staff that have not been authorised through the QMS should be investigated and are grounds for disciplinary action [4].

Details relating to the egg collection such as the date, operator and number of eggs must be recorded on either a paper document or directly onto a computer spreadsheet or database. If multiple work stations are used, the specific equipment should be recorded for traceability purposes. This form can and should be adapted to suit current laboratory requirements and as such is a 'living document'. The paperwork can keep up with any areas that may need to be tracked and the laboratory form will become bespoke to its respective IVF laboratory; a 'one size fits all' approach tends not to be appropriate, and the form would quickly evolve to suits the needs of the unit. Any adaptations should be approved by the laboratory/quality manager, a new version issued and the previous, now obsolete version, archived. Taking the example in Figure 10.3, for each cycle the document requires information regarding patient consent, viral screening results and the use of donor gametes. The dedicated scribing areas for donor codes, treatment types and information regarding previous cycles allow information to be accessed quickly by the embryologist to aid in decision making and communication, providing a more individualised approach to patient care and avoiding important information being overlooked. Tweaks to this paperwork should be acknowledged in the SOP and are an example of making marginal gains to ultimately improve patient satisfaction and overall clinic performance. All information that is recorded throughout the cycle is a permanent account that should be accurate, complete and traceable to a staff member. Following the cycle, the document should be appropriately filed and easily located for future use.

10.2.10 Process Validation

The process of collecting eggs must be validated to ensure that it provides the optimal outcome of obtaining an appropriate number of viable oocytes in line with current best practice [15]. The HFEA states that the process 'must not render the gametes or embryos clinically ineffective or harmful to the recipient' and creation of the SOP goes part way to satisfy this requirement [2]. The SOP is designed with influence from well-established procedures and data from previously published studies to explain why the process should be carried out a certain way. A literature search should inform on current practice and the safest, most efficient manner to collect the oocytes. Any improvements in egg collection methods or notable scientific discoveries regarding the handling of oocytes should be picked up through the literature search and considered when revising the process. By selecting only CE-marked consumables from accredited suppliers, servicing equipment regularly and assessing staff competence, the process can be assured as 'fit for purpose'. Once the process is implemented, retrospective analysis of outcome can either provide further reassurance or uncover flaws within the process that need to be addressed promptly. The process should be revalidated regularly to ensure that it is continually relevant.

10.3 Performance Monitoring

10.3.1 Key Performance Indicators

Key performance indicators (KPIs) are used to measure the success of the QMS that is in place, with 'live birth rate' and 'patient satisfaction' reflecting the performance of the unit overall. Individual staff KPIs can be analysed to reassure that all embryologists are working to the same standard, or to note where staff members may need extra support or further training. The personalised KPIs make it possible for embryologists to review their own practice and work to their own personal targets. Any improvements may then be shared with the team. The success of egg collection is reflected primarily in the fertilisation rate; however, other KPIs such as cleavage rate, percentage of embryos used for treatment and clinical pregnancy rate will also represent the success or failure of this procedure. It is not just in house that KPIs are monitored. The HFEA will assess clinic data and issue warnings (RBAT (risk-based assessment tool) alerts) where performance risks falling below the national average. Some variables such as patient age, body mass index or inherent oocyte quality cannot be controlled but will impact the KPIs and should be considered upon analysis. An expert meeting has established a consensus on reference values for KPIs within the IVF laboratory, with benchmarks ranging from 'competent' to 'aspirational goal' [16]. KPIs alert the laboratory manager to increasing or decreasing trends in performance, and declining success should be investigated to assess whether the trend can be attributed to a specific cause. An increase in success rates due to multiple marginal gains is the ultimate goal of quality improvement and should be celebrated as an indicator of a successful QMS.

10.3.2 Audit

Audit is performed to officially examine the documented records of the clinic to clarify how successfully the clinic's policies and processes are being adhered to. Audits can be carried out for any component of the whole system and at any time, and are not restricted to the laboratory. The outcome of the audit should be of benefit to the QMS by revealing areas of weakness within the system, and therefore offering opportunity for improvement. Audits relating to the egg collection procedure include:

Fresh IVF/ICSI lab report

Annotations	IDEAS	HFEA form sent	E-cycles book	Freeze letter	

		IVF ☐
Patient name:…………………………………	Partner name:…………………………………	ICSI ☐
DOB:…………………………………………	DOB:…………………………………………	SSR ☐
Hospital number:………………………	Hospital number:………………………	ET plan:
		CCG:

Previous cycles history	
Female infertility cause	Male infertility cause

BMI		D2 FSH		Protocol		Total FSH Dose	

If egg recipient; Egg donor code:	If egg sharing; Egg recip code:	If using donor sperm: Database checked? Reserved? Sperm donor code: Y N Y N
Double Witnessed:		If known donation; known gamete donor disclaimer: Donor Y N Recipient Y N

WT/WD	Eggs:	Training	Store: length:	Embryos:	Training	Store: length:	WP	ICSI	Tx w donor eggs ☐	Research
MT	Sperm:	Training	Store: length:	Embryos:	Training	Store length:	PP	ICSI	Tx w donor sperm ☐	PBR

DATE OF TEST	HIV	Hep B	Hep C	HTLV
Female:	☐ Neg ☐ Pos	☐ Neg ☐ Pos	☐ Neg ☐ Pos	☐ Neg ☐ Pos
Male:	☐ Neg ☐ Pos	☐ Neg ☐ Pos	☐ Neg ☐ Pos	☐ Neg ☐ Pos

ULTRASOUND GUIDED OOCYTE RETRIEVAL

Verbal Check: patient to paperwork OR dish ID to donor code	*Check screening in date* ☐
Date: ……………… Time: ……………	*Check no tubes in hot block / theatre:*
Embryologist: …………………………Initials……	Date: ……………… Time: ……………
Dr: …………………………………Initials……	Embryologist: …………………………Initials……
Nurse: ……………………………Initials……	Nurse: …………………………………Initials……

Side	Number of follicles	Number of eggs	*NEEDLE STICKER*
Left			
Right			
Total			DOUBLE SINGLE EXPIRY:

Time	Insem vol	DISH ONE		DISH TWO		DISH THREE	
	μl	Well 1	Well 2	Well 1	Well 2	Well 1	Well 2
Egg numbers							
Insem Witness							

Category	Embryology forms	Authorisation Date	06 09 18	Review Date	06 09 19
Title	Fresh IVF/ICSI lab report	Issue No	4	Author	
		Ref No	27	Page	1/4

Figure 10.3 Example of a laboratory form used for egg collection.

witnessing, competency review, temperature control review and documentation.

10.4 Summary

The QMS infiltrates every aspect of the fertility service, including oocyte collection, and, as such, should be considered as integral to the running of the clinic.

To truly perform at the highest standard, each component of egg collection must be scrutinised and its use justified through literature review, validation and continual in-house monitoring of success. By consistently engaging in QMS activities, improvements will be seen that ultimately lead to better outcomes for the clinic, its staff and its patients.

References

1. ESHRE Guideline Group on Good Practice in IVF Labs. Revised guidelines for good practice in IVF laboratories (2015). *Hum Reprod* 2016;**31**(4):685–6. doi: 10.1093/humrep/dew016

2. Human Fertilisation and Embryology Authority (HEFA). *Code of Practice*, 9th ed. London: HEFA, 2018. Available from: https://portal.hfea.gov.uk/knowledge-base/read-the-code-of-practice/

3. International Organization for Standardization (ISO). *Quality Management Principles*. Geneva: ISO, 2019. Available from: www.iso.org/publication/PUB100080.html

4. Mortimer ST, Mortimer D. *Quality and Risk Management in the IVF Laboratory*. Cambridge: Cambridge University Press, 2015.

5. Bontekoe S, Mantikou E. Low oxygen concentrations for embryo culture in assisted reproductive technologies. *Cochrane Database Syst Rev* 2012;7:CD008950. doi: 10.1002/14651858.CD008950.pub2

6. Pickering SJ. Transient cooling to room temperature can cause irreversible disruption of the meiotic spindle in the human oocyte. *Fertil Steril* 1990;**54** (1):102–8. doi: 10.1016/s0015-0282(16)53644-9

7. Swain JE. Decisions for the IVF laboratory: comparative analysis of embryo culture incubators. *Reprod Biomed Online* 2014;**28** (5):535–47. doi: 10.1016/j.rbmo.2014.01.004

8. Swain JE. Optimizing the culture environment in the IVF laboratory: impact of pH and buffer capacity on gamete and embryo quality. *Reprod Biomed Online* 2010;**21**(1):6–16. doi: 10.1016/j.rbmo.2010.03.012

9. European Commission. *The Rules Governing Medicinal Products in the European Union, Volume 4. EU Guidelines to Good Manufacturing Practice Medicinal Products for Human and Veterinary Use. Annex 1. Manufacture of Sterile Medicinal Products*. Brussels: European Commission, 2008. https://ec.europa.eu/health/sites/health/files/files/eudralex/vol-4/2008_11_25_gmp-an1_en.pdf

10. Morbeck D. Air quality in the assisted reproduction laboratory: a mini-review. *J Assist Reprod Genet* 2015;**32**(7):1019–24. doi: 10.1007/s10815-015-0535-x

11. Mortimer D, Cohen J. Cairo consensus on the IVF laboratory environment and air quality: report of an expert meeting. *Reprod Biomed Online* 2018;**36** (6):658–74. doi: 10.1016/j.rbmo.2018.02.005

12. Munch E. Lack of carbon air filtration impacts early embryo development. *J Assist Reprod Genet* 2015;**32**(7):1009–17. doi: 10.1007/s10815-015-0495-1

13. Critchlow D. Quality control in an in-vitro fertilization laboratory: use of human sperm survival studies. *Hum Reprod* 1989;**4**(5):545–9. doi: 10.1093/oxfordjournals.humrep.a136942

14. de los Santos MJ. Protocols for tracking and witnessing samples and patients in assisted reproductive technology. *Fertil Steril* 2013;**100**(6):1499–502. doi: 10.1016/j.fertnstert.2013.09.029

15. Hughes C, Association of Clinical Embryologists. Guidelines on good practice in clinical embryology laboratories *Hum Fertil (Camb)* 2012;**15**(4):174–89. doi: 10.3109/14647273.2012.747891

16. ESHRE Special Interest Group, Alpha Scientists in Reproductive Medicine. The Vienna consensus: report of an expert meeting on the development of ART laboratory performance indicators. *Reprod Biomed Online* 2017;**35** (5):494–510 doi: 10.1016/j.rbmo.2017.06.015.

Chapter 11

Morphological Assessment of Oocyte Quality

Basak Balaban, İpek Keles and Thomas Ebner

11.1 Introduction

Assessment of oocyte morphology and determination of its correlation with quality/viability and the clinical outcome is a difficult task, as the underlying mechanisms that change the appearance are multifactorial and complex. Optimal oocyte morphology is defined as an oocyte with spherical structure enclosed by a uniform zona pellucida (ZP), with a uniform translucent cytoplasm free of inclusions and a size-appropriate polar body (Pb) (Figure 11.1). However, oocytes at the metaphase II (MII) stage retrieved from patients after ovarian stimulation are known to show significant morphological variations that may affect the developmental competence and implantation potential of the derived embryo [1, 2].

More than half of oocytes collected can contain at least one morphological abnormality, and this may be correlated with the asynchrony between nuclear and

cytoplasmic maturation of the MII oocyte, playing an important role in its viability, and in the clinical outcome. Morphological variations of the oocyte may also result from other intrinsic factors such as age and genetic defects, or from extrinsic factors such as stimulation protocols, culture conditions and nutrition [1, 2]. Conflicting results are published in the literature regarding the effect of morphological variations of the oocyte on embryo development and implantation.

This chapter will review the correlation of morphological abnormalities of the MII oocyte and clinical outcome, and the effect on genetic disorders, and will discuss the predictive value of specific abnormalities and examine whether any of these parameters can be utilised in scoring systems applied in in vitro fertilisation (IVF) laboratories.

Morphological abnormalities of the oocyte will be discussed as two different subgroups: cytoplasmic abnormalities and extracytoplasmic abnormalities [1–3]

11.2 Cytoplasmic Abnormalities

Cytoplasmic abnormalities of MII oocytes include different types and degrees of cytoplasmic granulations (slightly diffused or excessive whole/centrally located granulation) and the appearance of refractile bodies, smooth endoplasmic reticulum clusters (SERCs) or vacuolisation in the ooplasm. Detection of cytoplasmic variations was first termed cytoplasmic dysmorphism in the early 1990s, and since then has been used as a selection method to assess the viability and implantation potential of the derived embryos.

11.2.1 Morphological Appearance of the Cytoplasm

Although the appearance of the cytoplasm was considered a potential predictive factor for the success of

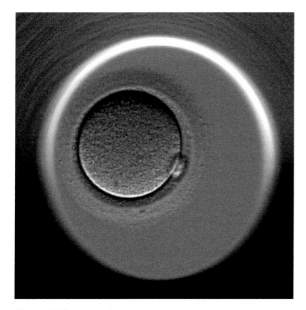

Figure 11.1 A normal mature oocyte.

clinical outcome, different definitions and grouping of multiple morphological features in various published studies make comparative analysis difficult. The terms that have been used in the literature are: dark cytoplasm, dark cytoplasm–granular cytoplasm, dark cytoplasm with slight granulation, dark granular appearance of the cytoplasm and diffused cytoplasmic granularity [4, 5]. The high subjectivity of the definition of these types of granulations in various laboratories means that there is limited predictive value for the clinical outcome. Despite the fact that the majority of clinical trials examining the effect of dark granular cytoplasm as an individual feature showed no detrimental effect on the viability of the derived embryo [4, 6], and was even perhaps associated with higher fertilisation when compared with oocytes with total absence of granularity, conflicting results were also published [5]. Variations in these publications may be correlated with the subjectivity of the definition, as diffused slight cytoplasmic granularity, also called dark cytoplasm, can be ill defined and could differ by different modulation of the optical path in phase-contrast microscopy in various laboratories. Homogeneity of the cytoplasm is expected (Figure 11.1); however, the biological significance of non-homogeneity is unknown and, based on current evidence, it may simply represent variability between oocytes rather than a dysmorphism of developmental significance [1].

11.2.2 Centrally Located Granulation of the Cytoplasm

Condensed granulation that is centrally located within the cytoplasm with a clear border (Figure 11.2) is unlike the various degrees of diffused granulation described above as it is easily distinguishable with a significant darker appearance than normal cytoplasm and is clearly visible by any modulation type of the optical path in different phase-contrast microscopies. It was first defined by Serhal et al. with a detrimental effect on the outcome of intracytoplasmic sperm injection (ICSI) [7], and was later named centrally located granular cytoplasm (CLGC) by Kahraman et al. [8]. CLGC is a rare morphological feature of the oocyte that is diagnosed as a large, dark, spongy, granular area in the cytoplasm, and the severity is based on both the diameter of the granular area and the depth of the lesion.

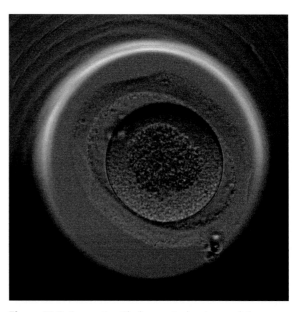

Figure 11.2 An oocyte with dense cytoplasmic granulation.

Although fertilisation rate and embryo quality were not affected in the study by Kahraman et al. [8], the risk of poor ongoing pregnancy correlating with high aneuploidy (52.3%) and abortion rates (54.5%) was associated with the transfer of embryos derived from oocytes with severe CLGC. A study by Meriano et al. [9] defined CLGC oocytes as organelle clustering and determined that this particular abnormality is the only repetitive dysmorphism in consecutive cycles and is a negative predictor of pregnancy and implantation rates in intracytoplasmic injection cycles. It has also been demonstrated that MII oocytes that exhibited severe cytoplasmic disorganisation have a lower intracytoplasmic pH and ATP content, as well as increased incidence of aneuploidy and chromosomal scattering, findings that were later confirmed by Kahraman et al. [8]. Yakin et al. [10] also showed that the embryos that were derived from oocytes with severe cytoplasmic abnormalities where CLGC oocytes were included had a higher rate of aneuploidy (60.0%) compared with a group of embryos derived from oocytes with a normal morphological appearance (41.9%). However, the results were not statistically different, most likely based on insufficient numbers of embryos included in the comparison. The same group demonstrated that cryopreserved day 3 cleavage-stage embryos derived from oocytes with severe cytoplasmic abnormalities where CLGC oocytes comprised the majority of the

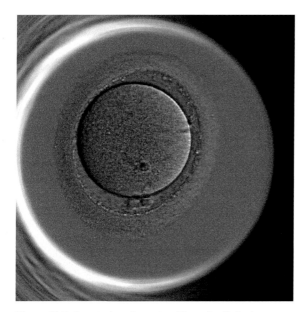

Figure 11.3 A metaphase II oocyte with a refractile body.

cytoplasmic abnormalities are examined jointly, so data on the individual predictive value of refractile bodies on clinical outcome are limited. Evidence based on data over the years shows conflicting results for the effect of cytoplasmic inclusions on fertilisation rates, embryo quality and implantation rates. Rienzi et al. showed that refractile bodies do not detrimentally affect fertilisation and normal pronuclear morphology rates [5]. In contrast, Otsuki et al. reported decreased fertilisation and embryo development [11]. It is likely that conflicting results may be correlated to the factors that are still unknown, and one possible confounding factor could be the differing diameters of refractile bodies. Only one study in the literature has examined precisely the relationship between the sizes of the refractile bodies and the developmental competence of oocytes, and found that lipofuscin inclusions were associated with reduced fertilisation and unfavourable blastocyst development only when their diameter is greater than 5 μm [11]. This study also showed that the size of refractile bodies is not correlated with the age of the women, or with different stimulation protocols, and that the embryo developmental outcome was not significantly affected by stimulation regimes [11]. These authors found that the ageing of oocytes during inactive phases of oogenesis may not be involved with lipofuscinogenesis; instead, the accumulation of lipofuscin may occur during the growth phase of the oocytes when dominant follicles are being recruited into the pre-ovulatory pathway [11]. The occurrence of large lipofuscin bodies in normal ageing may also be related to conditions of the developing ovarian follicles, such as perifollicular blood circulation and follicular fluid composition. Other explanations can be related to oxidative stress, proteolytic degradation or lipid metabolism as a source of energy supply. Further research is needed to investigate whether any of these possibilities are involved in causing the refractile bodies that are mainly correlated with lipofuscinogenesis in human oocytes.

experimental group had a significantly lower cryosurvival rate. If these embryos survived, they had lower rates of blastocyst formation, and none of the blastocysts obtained was of good quality or was able to successfully complete the hatching process [4]. Based on the evidence, it is important to inform patients about such morphological defects of the MII oocyte, and the reduced implantation outcome and increased risk of aneuploidy with the resultant embryos [1].

11.2.3 Refractile Bodies

Refractile bodies are cytoplasmic inclusions that can be dark incorporations, fragments, spots, dense granules, lipid droplets or lipofuscin (Figure 11.3). Transmission electron microscopy studies and Schmorl staining have shown that refractile bodies greater than 5 μm show the conventional morphology of lipofuscin inclusions consisting of a mixture of lipids and dense granular materials. Lipofuscin bodies in human oocytes can be detected throughout meiotic maturation (in the germinal vesicle (GV) and through metaphase I (MI) and MII), a situation that is different from other cytoplasmic abnormalities in humans, such as SERCs, which appear only in mature (MII stage) oocytes [11].

The average diameter of a recognisable refractile body under bright-field microscopy is approximately 10 μm. As in the majority of published articles,

11.2.4 Vacuoles

Vacuoles are membrane-bound cytoplasmic inclusions filled with fluid that is virtually identical to the perivitelline space (PVS) liquid (Figure 11.4). Their sizes and numbers may vary, and it is assumed that these vacuoles arise either spontaneously or by fusion of pre-existing vesicles derived from smooth

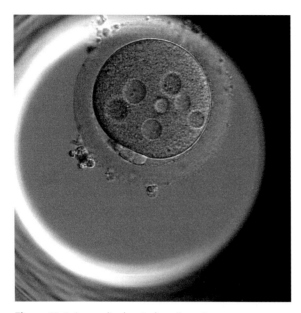

Figure 11.4 A vacuolised metaphase II oocyte.

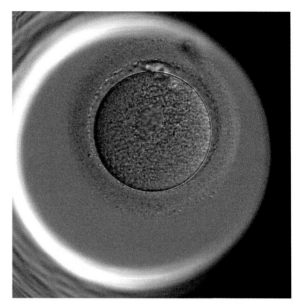

Figure 11.5 An oocyte with a centrally located smooth endoplasmic reticulum.

endoplasmic reticulum (SER) and/or Golgi apparatus, or both [12].

The incidence of vacuoles in MII oocytes varies from 3.1% to 12.4%. However, multiple vacuolisation occurs less frequently, in approximately 1–1.5% [13]. Ebner et al. reported a significantly decreased fertilisation rate with oocytes containing single vacuoles (51.6%) and multiple vacuoles (43.8%) compared with oocytes without vacuoles (65.3%) [13]. Rienzi et al. also demonstrated a significantly reduced fertilisation rate for vacuolated oocytes; however, pronuclear morphology and embryo quality were not detrimentally affected [5]. Only one study carried out subgroup analysis examining the effect of the size of the vacuoles on fertilisation rates and found that the group of oocytes that fertilised normally contained vacuoles that were less than 9.8 ± 3.7 μm in diameter [13], a value that was significantly smaller than the diameter of vacuoles in the unfertilised oocytes (17.6 ± 9.0 μm). A cut-off value of 14 μm for vacuole diameter was noted above which fertilisation did not occur. This study showed that a larger vacuole or multiple vacuoles may have a much more detrimental effect on the oocyte than a small vacuole, because a larger portion of the cytoskeleton (e.g. microtubules) cannot function as it is supposed to. It has been suggested that large vacuoles might displace the MII spindle from its polar position, resulting in fertilisation failure, cleavage abnormalities, abnormal cytokinesis pattern or various combinations of these effects. Although the presence of a few small vacuoles (5–10 μm in diameter) that are fluid filled but transparent is unlikely to be of biological consequence, observation of large vacuoles greater than 14 μm in diameter should be noted [1]. As well as the decrease in fertilisation rates, it has also been shown that blastocyst formation, good-quality blastocysts and hatching blastocyst rates can significantly decrease after ICSI of vacuolated oocytes. The percentage of aneuploid embryos can also be affected by the use of vacuolated oocytes (41.9%) compared with embryos that are derived from oocytes with normal morphology (60.0%) [10]. Vacuolisation in MII oocytes can also decrease cryosurvival rates and subsequent embryonic development of the derived cryopreserved embryos [4].

11.2.5 SERCs

The presence of SERCs in the cytoplasm of MII oocytes is one of the most important cytoplasmic defects and demands careful examination (Figure 11.5). A correlation between the presence of SERCs in MII oocytes, and the clinical outcome was first published by Otsuki et al. [14]. They reported that in approximately 10% of cycles, cytoplasmic localisation of translucent disc-like structures, of a similar sized to pronuclei, exist at the MII stage of human oocytes after the denuding procedure for ICSI. Although this incidence varied between 5% and 7% in the literature, it is likely that the number of oocytes with SERCs is underestimated because it has been shown by transmission electron microscopic analysis that there are at least three forms of SERCs: large (18 μm) and medium (10–17 μm), which can be classified by light microscopy, and small (2–9 μm), which are not visible under the conditions used in clinical embryology laboratories for examination. SERCs can easily be distinguished from fluid-filled vacuoles because they are not separated from the rest of the ooplasmic volume by a membrane and are seen as translucent disc-like structures. Although the mechanism responsible for SERCs is still unknown, there are some human and animal studies suggesting that it could be correlated to functional and structural alterations of the SER during oocyte maturation, such as an increase in the sensitivity of the IP3 receptor for calcium ions (Ca^{2+}), increased storage of Ca^{2+} that is released during oscillation, changes in the structure from a sheet-like form to a spherical form in starfish oocytes, and distribution of the SER in mouse oocytes. In human oocytes, the localisation of mobilisable Ca^{2+} was detected in the small vesicles beneath the plasma membrane of SER. Otsuki et al. compared the clinical outcome of patients with oocytes containing SERCs and patients with retrieved oocytes without SERCs, and examined whether any confounding parameters such as stimulation methods or hormonal levels could affect the outcome [14]. Fertilisation rate and embryo quality were not detrimentally affected; however, significantly lower clinical pregnancy and implantation and significantly higher biochemical pregnancy were observed for SERC-positive cycles. Due to the limited number of samples tested, no significant differences were found between the study groups when stimulation protocols were compared. However, the number of SERC-positive oocytes obtained by the short protocol was about three times larger than that by the long protocol. Serum oestradiol levels on the day of human chorionic gonadotropin administration were significantly higher in SERC-positive cycles. This study clearly showed that the viability of an embryo is significantly reduced by the presence of SERCs. Even if the embryo is derived from an oocyte without any clusters, its implantation potential is detrimentally affected if the oocyte is from a cohort of oocytes where at least one oocyte has clusters. Together with the viability of the derived

embryos, the most important issue with the presence of SERCs is neonatal safety based on evidence in the literature. In the Otsuki study, in the one pregnancy derived from gametes with an SER defect, the baby was diagnosed with Beckwith–Wiedemann syndrome [14].

Ebner et al. showed that the occurrence of SERCs is significantly related to a longer duration and higher dosage of the stimulation [15]. Fertilisation and blastocyst formation rate were significantly lower for oocytes with SERCs when compared with oocytes without SERCs. The take-home baby rate was significantly lower in the group with SERCs, and the miscarriage rate was significantly higher in the same group of patients. Pregnancies in women with affected gametes had a significantly higher incidence of obstetric problems. The birth weight of babies born in the group with SERCs was significantly lower, and there were two unexplained neonatal deaths reported in the group with affected gametes, whereas there were no deaths reported in the group without SERCs. The malformation rate was similar in both groups, with one case of diaphragmatic hernia reported in the group with SERCs. These similar findings reported by Otsuki et al. [14] and Ebner et al. [15] support the idea that this phenomenon is the manifestation of an intrinsic oocyte defect caused by suboptimal ovarian stimulation, and perhaps as a result of overstimulation. Following other studies reporting multiple malformations and ventricular septal defects after the transfer of embryos originating from oocytes with SERCs, it was strongly recommended on the ALPHA-ESHRE Istanbul consensus document that oocytes with this feature should not be inseminated, and even that the sibling oocytes should be examined carefully [1].

Despite the fact that controversial results reported on neonatal outcome over the years suggest that the fate of babies born from oocytes with this feature should be very carefully evaluated and reported, a recent review by Ferreux et al. successfully clarified the current situation about this severe cytoplasmic abnormality [16]. Although the ALPHA-ESHRE Istanbul consensus document recommended not injecting/inseminating oocytes with SERCs due to the adverse neonatal outcomes reported, recent clinical studies have shown promising results, with healthy babies born. Based on this recent literature, Ferreux et al. recommend that all mature oocytes should be inseminated and embryos originating from oocytes without SERCs should be preferably transferred, even if they come from a cohort of oocytes with SERCs. When only embryos deriving from oocytes with SER remain, the couple should be provided with appropriate information concerning the available literature data on the topic in order to help them make a decision [1, 16].

11.3 Extracytoplasmic Abnormalities

A variety of extracytoplasmic anomalies exist that in part negatively influence fertilisation (consistency and thickness of the ZP, Pb1 decay and debris within the PVS), blastulation (thickness of ZP, Pb1 fragmentation) and pregnancy (thickness of ZP, Pb1 morphology and debris in the PVS). The characteristics of the ZP and PVS are most probably associated with the health of the developing follicle, such as its vascularisation and oxygen content. Any disturbance during growth might severely alter oocyte morphology resulting in a pool of gametes with different prognoses.

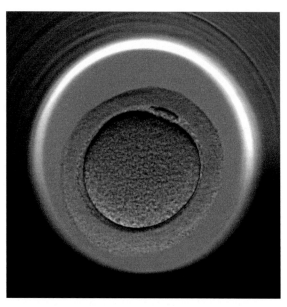

Figure 11.6 An extremely thick zona pellucida.

11.3.1 Dysmorphic ZP

As a result of the mutual dependence between somatic cells (e.g. cumulus cells) and the egg, it is likely that any disturbance negatively affecting the follicle will have a comparable impact on the oocyte itself. Among the conceivable changes in oocyte performance, it is possible that the secretion or patterning of the ZP from the secondary follicle onwards could be altered or interrupted [17]. This could either result in dysmorphism that can be seen under a light microscope (Figures 11.6 and 11.7) or in more subtle changes of the three-dimensional structure of the ZP. Normally, four ZP proteins build up the three-dimensional matrix of the outer protective shell, and the most severe form of impaired growth of the ZP is its complete absence.

In humans, a defect in gene expression was shown to cause a failure in the glycoprotein matrix, even though the ovum itself showed intact corona cells [18]. In such rare cases, the ovum fails to fertilise in conventional IVF. In ICSI, there is a considerable risk of exposing the gametes to mechanical stress during the denudation process. Studies have shown that, in patients with ZP-free eggs, pregnancies can be achieved by simply leaving the coronal cell layer attached, as it acts as a supporting structure keeping the oocyte in shape during injection. [18].

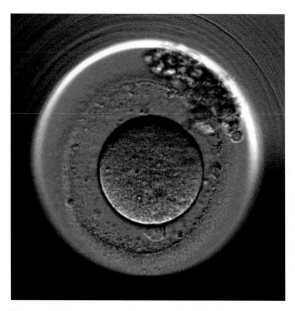

Figure 11.7 An extremely thin zona pellucida and large perivitelline space.

From conventional IVF, it is known that a thicker ZP (e.g. >20 μm) is associated with lower fertilisation rates. This has been linked to patient and stimulation parameters. In ICSI, however, a thicker ZP does not interfere with subsequent fertilisation or with implantation, as assisted hatching can be applied.

The multilaminar structure of the ZP can also be analysed quantitatively using polarised light microscopy [19]. Although variation exists in the thickness of ZP layers around individual eggs and among members of a cohort, it is evident that the inner layer is the most dominant part of the ZP [17, 19]. It has been reported that the birefringence of the inner layer is directly proportional to its thickness [17, 20].

Clinical studies investigating the relationship between ZP birefringence (inner layer) and pre-implantation development suggest that embryo quality, blastocyst formation and clinical outcome can be impaired by low birefringence scores [17, 20, 21].

11.3.2 Discoloration

Irrespective of the actual thickness of the ZP, ovarian stimulation sometimes generates gametes showing a ZP that appears dark or brownish under a light microscope. Mostly, the egg itself is affected. It is reported that the presence of a discoloured ZP is a common phenomenon, occurring at a rate at 9.5–25.7% [4, 22]. However, it is not completely clear that dark or brown zonae/oocytes occur for the same reasons. These oocytes were termed 'brown eggs' because they were found to be dark with a thick ZP, a rather small PVS (sometimes filled with debris) and granular cytoplasm. Esfandiari et al. prospectively compared the outcome of brown gametes with that of gametes of normal appearance [23]. Although the ZP in discoloured eggs was thicker than that of control gametes, in conventional IVF, the fertilisation rate was similar. The same was true for fertilisation after ICSI, embryo quality, implantation rate and clinical pregnancy rate. However, because of the thick ZP, brown oocytes were subjected to laser-assisted hatching significantly more often than the control group.

11.3.3 Shape Anomalies

Even if the thickness or colour of the ZP has no visible defect, it is not automatic that the shape of the gametes is spherical. Indeed, there is evidence that extremely ovoid eggs exist. Such gametes have been shown to be fertilisable and may lead to the birth of a healthy baby. However, a major problem with these reports is that the degree of the shape anomaly was not quantified and rather imprecise descriptions have been given (e.g. cucumber shaped).

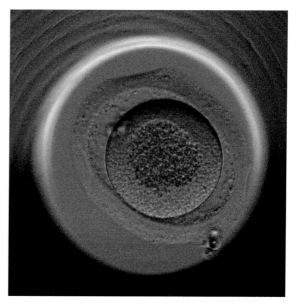

Figure 11.8 A spherical-shaped oocyte with an ovoid zona pellucida showing centrally located granulation.

Ebner et al. successfully measured ovoid oocytes and calculated a roundness index (RI, length divided by width) [24]. Actually, two indices were determined to assess whether the whole oocyte was affected (showing an ovoid ooplasm and ZP) or only the ZP was of ovoid shape (with the ooplasm being perfectly round) (Figures 11.8 and 11.9). Special care was taken to detect splitting of the innermost ZP layer that might keep the ooplasm as a round shape (while the ZP is ovoid). This latter dysmorphism was shown to be associated with implantation failure [17].

The degree of shape anomaly was not correlated to fertilisation or embryo quality [25]. Interestingly, two types of cleavage pattern were observed on day 2. Either ovoid gametes cleaved normally like a tetrahedron (a cross-wise arrangement of four cells with three blastomeres lying side by side) or, if the ovoid ZP failed to exert its shaping function, they resulted in a rather flat array of four blastomeres. Because the abnormal pattern reduces the number of cell-to-cell contact points from six to five or four, compaction and blastulation of the corresponding embryos may be delayed [24].

Two possible mechanisms may account for the occurrence of ovoid oocytes. Mechanical stress during oocyte puncture, denudation processes, or both could deform the egg. This unwanted occurrence would create ovoid gametes with both the ooplasm and ZP

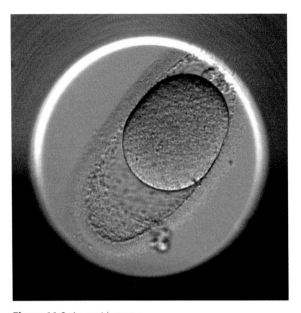

Figure 11.9 An ovoid oocyte.

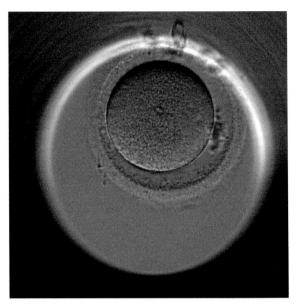

Figure 11.10 A metaphase II oocyte with a large perivitelline space.

being affected. In these artificially damaged gametes, a tendency towards recovery within a day has been suggested [24]. Thus, for the majority of ovoid ova, it can be assumed that the deformation is a pre-existing anomaly generated during maturation within the follicle.

11.3.4 PVS

The size of the PVS is closely related to the maturational phase of the oocyte. Whereas at GV stage (prophase I), expansion of the PVS is minimal, it begins to increase after resumption of meiosis. In detail, at MI, the PVS can clearly be detected and after completion of maturation (MII) its full size is reached.

Several studies have noted that up to 50% of all ova show a large PVS [5]. In oocytes with a larger PVS (Figure 11.10), a lower fertilisation rate was observed compared with gametes with a normal-sized gap. This is more or less in line with the results of Rienzi et al. who showed that a large PVS is detrimental to fertilisation and zygote morphology [6]. Interestingly, patient parameters such as female age and indication did not seem to influence PVS performance but the ratio of oestradiol to testosterone (and to progesterone) did [25].

Data from in vitro- and in vivo-matured oocytes indicate that a large PVS may be ascribed to

overmature eggs [26]. Such eggs have shrunk in relation to the ZP, presenting a large gap in between. A large PVS would also occur if a larger portion of cytoplasm is extruded together with the haploid chromosomal set during first Pb formation. This would result in a large first Pb and a large PVS.

11.3.5 First Pb Morphology

For a long time it was thought that first Pb (Pb1) extrusion marks the completion of nuclear maturation ending in a MII oocyte. However, by using polarised light microscopy, it was demonstrated that some oocytes showing a Pb1 were actually in telophase I and not in MII [27]. Otsuki et al. found a chromosome aggregation phase, which occurred not only from GV breakdown to MI but also from telophase I to MII [28]. If ICSI is performed, although the chromosomes are unaligned, it may result in failed fertilisation or three pronuclear zygotes due to abnormal chromosomal segregation.

Based primarily on this biological hypothesis, several studies in the literature have discussed the beneficial effect of careful examination of the meiotic spindle presence and especially its morphological features prior to ICSI to improve fertilisation rates, embryo quality and clinical outcome. Due to the fact that observation of the meiotic spindle requires polarised microscopy, like ZP birefringence evaluation, and that accurate visualisation of the meiotic spindle is highly sensitive to physical and chemical procedures carried out in the embryology laboratory, routine examination of the spindle prior to ICSI for all cases remains a debate. Future morphokinetic studies will provide more information on how the dynamic changes of the ZP and meiotic spindle within hours of the in vitro maturation period prior to ICSI may affect the clinical outcome and will help to understand the extent to which deep analysis of the ZP and meiotic spindle features could be used as objective biomarkers of oocyte quality [29].

The impact of Pb1 morphology on clinical outcome had always been a discussion based on controversial clinical results reported. Although some Pb1s in humans remain intact for more than 20 hours after ovulation, they generally have a shorter life span. Taking this time dependency into consideration, it might be hypothesised that Pb1 morphology provides adequate information on the actual post-ovulatory age of the corresponding egg [26].

Apparently, the benefit of selecting oocytes according to the morphology of the Pb1 is somewhat reduced with increasing time span between ovulation induction and ICSI, because studies with different schedules could not find a relationship between the constitution of the Pb1 and subsequent ICSI outcome [30]. In these data sets, the percentage of oocytes with fragmented Pbs (Figure 11.11) was higher [30, 31] than that reported in the work of Ebner et al. [22] in which Pbs were scored 2 hours after collection. This is in line with the finding that of all intact Pb1s, 13% were already fragmented at a second inspection 3 hours later [31]. For practical reasons and in order to minimise the risk of oocyte ageing in vitro, ICSI should be finished within 12 hours of retrieval [32]. Future studies on the dynamics of Pb1 fragmentation may demonstrate better whether this morphological feature can be used as an objective biomarker of oocyte quality and viability.

It is suggested that a large Pb1 impacts outcome significantly (Figure 11.12). When large Pb1s were extruded, embryos with multinucleated blastomeres were significantly more frequent than in all other Pb1 classes. It has been postulated that the extrusion of an abnormally large Pb1 is due to dislocation of the meiotic spindle, as this would in part explain the observed impact on fertilisation and embryo development [5, 22, 30].

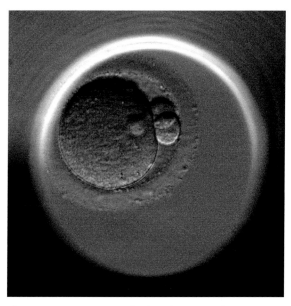

Figure 11.11 An oocyte with a large fragmented first polar body.

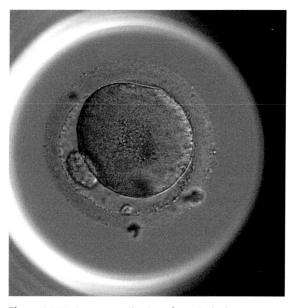

Figure 11.12 An oocyte with a large first polar body.

11.3.6 Debris in the PVS

Sometimes it is difficult to distinguish between heavily fragmented Pb1s and debris within the PVS. Two hypotheses have been proposed in order to explain the origin of the latter dysmorphism. One hypothesis is derived from ultrastructural data indicating the presence of an extracellular matrix comprised of granules and filaments in the space between the oolemma and ZP because the matrix is identical to that found between cumulus cells and the corona radiata. The second hypothesis is based on the existence of coronal cell processes passing the ZP and reaching the egg early in maturation. It is suggested that after withdrawal of these processes, some remnants remain within the PVS. Fertilisation rate, cleavage rate and embryo quality were found to be unaffected by the presence of coarse granules in the PVS; however, rates of implantation and pregnancy seem to be affected, because transfer of embryos derived from PVS granule-free oocytes increased the implantation rate by 5% and the pregnancy rate by 21% [33].

11.4 Summary

The final end point for evaluating morphological abnormalities of MII oocytes is to be able to correlate them with oocyte quality and viability, and thus increase the overall efficiency of human-assisted reproduction in terms of clinical success and safety of offspring. High heterogeneity of the published material and subjectivity of the evaluation of morphological deviations of MII oocytes may only provide limited take-home messages on the predictive value of outcome parameters for successful results. The most recent meta-analysis examining the clinical results of 40 relevant articles on previously described extracytoplasmic and cytoplasmic abnormalities showed that there was no clear tendency to a general increase in predictive value of morphological features and that these contradicting findings underline the importance of more intensive and coordinated research that would lead to more objective criteria with better predictive value to determine the viability of derived embryos [34]. Rapidly developing continuous research on new biomarkers of oocyte quality may perhaps be used in addition or as an alternative to morphological assessment in the future; however, the current limited predictive value of morphology should not be underestimated considering that it remains the sole method for selection until a more effective technology can substitute for it in routine practice in clinical IVF laboratories. Beyond the predictive value of oocyte morphology, it must not be forgotten that information linking dysmorphism with genetic disorders is of great value as these disorders are directly correlated with the health of the offspring

in assisted reproductive technology applications [35]. According to a common hypothesis, the vast majority of extracytoplasmic anomalies occur late in maturation because they are associated with fertilisation and developmental failure rather than with aneuploidy (e.g. giant eggs). However, evidence-based data clearly demonstrate that some specific severe cytoplasmic defects are correlated with chromosomal aneuploidy and genetic disorders, as described above. It is obvious that some anomalies, for example, so-called giant eggs [36] with an almost double-sized diameter, show a diploid chromosomal set that contributes to digynic triploidy. Other studies analysed embryos genetically according to their Pb classes [37]. No correlation was observed between Pb shape and genetic constitution; however, the only Pb group bearing a theoretical risk of chromosomal disorder, considering the larger volume of ooplasm in large Pbs, was not analysed.

11.5 Future Directions

Despite various novel technologies being described in the literature to select viable oocytes in assisted reproductive technology, current strategies for assessment in routine clinical laboratory work rely primarily on morphological parameters with the awareness of its limited accuracy for determining viability [38]. As metabolism is the key determinant of cell survival, technologies that are able to non-invasively assess metabolic parameters could be exploited in the near future to improve our understanding of oocyte viability. Recent studies discussing the molecular methods and omics technologies for selection of the ideal oocyte will assist us in understanding the mystery of oocyte health and viability, and hopefully, in the future, will be adaptable in routine clinical practice for oocyte selection [39].

Other promising technologies for objective oocyte viability assessment may involve the efficient analysis of somatic cells surrounding the oocyte, the cumulus cells, as the intimate relationship between these cells and the oocyte allows bidirectional communication, which is essential for regulation of oocyte growth and acquisition of developmental competence through nuclear and cytoplasmic maturation [40].

Use of biomechanical properties as a potential marker of cellular health would be another interesting area to explore in the future, as promising results are being demonstrated in the literature [41].

Perhaps the best approach to select viable oocytes that would lead to healthy offspring will involve the utilisation of all these technologies in a joint manner that could additionally be combined with kinetics as well as genetic markers [42].

It is unquestionable that the ideal method of oocyte selection in the future should be non-invasive, inexpensive, objective in terms of predicting oocyte viability and able to be incorporated into embryology workflow with minimal disruption.

Future non-invasive approaches should be a major research goal that will enable us to monitor the consequences of different stimulation protocols and identify the underlying mechanisms by which they influence oocyte quality. The relationship between the effect of ovarian stimulation protocols on oocyte quality, including the morphological characteristics of the oocyte with its biological and functional properties, should be elucidated non-invasively, thus providing us with the opportunity to devise novel stimulation strategies for the optimisation of oocyte quality [43, 44].

References

1. ALPHA Scientists in Reproductive Medicine, ESHRE Special Interest Group of Embryology. The Istanbul consensus workshop on embryo assessment: proceedings of an expert meeting. *Reprod Biomed Online* 2011;**22** (6):632–46. doi: 10.1093/humrep/der037

2. Rienzi L, Balaban B, Ebner T, Mandelbaum J. The oocyte. *Hum Reprod* 2012;**27**:i2–21. doi: 10.1093/humrep/des200

3. Balaban B, Urman B. Effect of oocyte morphology on embryo development and implantation. *Reprod Biomed Online* 2006;**12** (5):608–15. doi: 10.1016/s1472-6483(10)61187-x

4. Balaban B, Ata B, Isiklar A, Yakin K, Urman B. Severe cytoplasmic abnormalities of the oocyte decrease cryosurvival and subsequent embryonic development of cryopreserved embryos. *Hum Reprod* 2008;**23** (8):1778–85. doi: 10.1093/humrep/den127

5. Rienzi L, Ubaldi FM, Lacobelli M, et al. Significance of metaphase II human oocyte morphology on ICSI outcome. *Fertil Steril* 2008;**90** (5):1692–700. doi: 10.1016/j.fertnstert.2007.09.024

6. Balaban B, Urman B, Sertac A, et al. Oocyte morphology does not affect fertilization rate, embryo quality and implantation rate after intracytoplasmic sperm injection.

Hum Reprod 1998;**13**(12);3431–3. doi: 10.1093/humrep/13.12.3431.

7. Serhal PF, Ranieri DM, Kinis A, et al. Oocyte morphology predicts outcome of intracytoplasmic sperm injection. *Hum Reprod* 1997;**12**(6):1267–70. doi: 10.1093/humrep/12.6.1267

8. Kahraman S, Yakin K, Dönmez E, et al. Relationship between granular cytoplasm of oocytes and pregnancy outcome following intracytoplasmic sperm injection. *Hum Reprod* 2000;**15**(11):2390–3. doi: 10.1093/humrep/15.11.2390

9. Meriano JM, Alexis J, Visram-Zaver S, Cruz M, Casper RF. Tracking of oocyte dysmorphisms for ICSI patients may prove relevant to the outcome in subsequent patient cycles. *Hum Reprod* 2001;**16**(10):2118–23. doi: 10.1093/humrep/16.10.2118

10. Yakin K, Balaban B, Isiklar A, Urman B. Oocyte dysmorphism is not associated with aneuploidy in the developing embryo. *Fertil Steril* 2006;**88**(4):811–16. doi: 10.1016/j.fertnstert.2006.12.031

11. Otsuki J, Nagai Y, Chiba K. Lipofuscin bodies in human oocytes as an indicator of oocyte quality. *J Assist Reprod Genet* 2007;**24**(7):263–70. doi: 10.1007/s10815-007-9130-0

12. El Shafie M, Sousa M, Windt ML, Kruger TF. Ultrastructure of human oocytes: a transmission electron microscopic view. In: *An Atlas of the Ultrastructure of Human Oocytes. A Guide for*

Assisted Reproduction. New York, London: Parthenon Publishing, 2000; 151–71.

13. Ebner T, Moser M, Sommergruber M, et al. Occurrence and developmental consequences of vacuoles throughout preimplantation development. *Fertil Steril* 2005;**83** (6):1635–40. doi: 10.1016/j.fertnstert.2005.02.009

14. Otsuki J, Okada A, Morimoto K, Nagai Y, Kubo H. The relationship between pregnancy outcome and smooth endoplasmic reticulum clusters in MII human oocytes. *Hum Reprod* 2004;**17** (7):1591–7. doi: 10.1093/humrep/deh258

15. Ebner T, Moser M, Shebl O, Sommergruber M, Tews G. Prognosis of oocytes showing aggregation of smooth endoplasmic reticulum. *Reprod Biomed Online* 2008;**16** (1):113–18. doi: 10.1016/s1472-6483(10)60563-9

16. Ferreux L, Sallem A, Chargui A, et al. Is it time to reconsider how to manage oocytes affected by smooth endoplasmic reticulum aggregates? *Hum Reprod* 2019;**34** (4):591–600. doi:10.1093/humrep/dez010.

17. Shen Y, Stalf T, Mehnert C, Eichenlaub-Ritter U, Tinneburg HR. High magnitude of light retardation by the zona pellucida is associated with conception cycles. *Hum Reprod* 2005;**20** (6):1596–606. doi: 10.1093/humrep/deh811

18. Stanger JD, Stevenson K, Lakmaker A, Woolcott R. Pregnancy following fertilization of zona-free, coronal cell intact human ova: case report. *Hum Reprod* 2001;**16**(1):164–7. doi: 10.1093/humrep/16.1.164

19. Pelletier C, Keefe D, Trimarchi JR. Noninvasive polarized light microscopy quantitatively distinguishes the multilaminar structure of the zona pellucida of living human eggs and embryos. *Fertil Steril* 2004;**81** (Suppl. 1):850–6. doi: 10.1016/j.fertnstert.2003.09.033.

20. Montag M., Schimming T, Zhou C. Oral validation of an automatic scoring system for prognostic qualitative zona imaging in human oocytes. *Hum Reprod* 2007;**22**(Suppl. 1):i11.

21. Ebner T, Balaban B, Moser M, et al. Automatic user-independent zona pellucida imaging at the oocyte stage allows for the prediction of preimplantation development. *Fertil Steril* 2010;**94** (3):913–20. doi:10.1016/j.fertnstert.2009.03.106. Epub 2009 May 12.

22. Ebner T., Yaman C., Moser M, et al. Prognostic value of first polar body morphology on fertilization rate and embryo quality in intracytoplasmic sperm injection. *Hum Reprod* 2000;**15** (2):427–30. doi: 10.1093/humrep/15.2.427

23. Esfandiari N, Burjaq H, Gotlieb L, et al. Brown oocytes: implications for assisted reproductive technology. *Fertil Steril* 2006;**86** (5):1522–5. doi: 10.1016/j.fertnstert.2006.03.056

24. Ebner T, Shebl O, Moser M, Sommergruber M, Tews G, Developmental fate of ovoid oocytes. *Hum Reprod* 2008;**23** (1):62–6. doi: 10.1093/humrep/dem280

25. Xia P, Younglai EV. Relationship between steroid concentrations in ovarian follicular fluid and oocyte morphology in patients undergoing intracytoplasmic sperm injection (ICSI) treatment. *J Reprod Fertil* 2000;**118**:229–33. doi: 10.1530/jrf.0.1180229

26. Miao YL, Kikuchi K, Sun QY, Schatten H. Oocyte aging: cellular and molecular changes, developmental potential and reversal possibility. *Hum Reprod Update* 2009;**15**(5):573–85. doi: 10.1093/humupd/dmp014

27. Montag M, Schimming T, van der Ven H. Spindle imaging in human oocytes: the impact of the meiotic cell cycle. *Reprod Biomed Online* 2006;**12**(4):442–6. doi: 10.1016/s1472-6483(10)61996-7

28. Otsuki J, Nagai Y. A phase of chromosome aggregation during meiosis in human oocytes. *Reprod Biomed Online* 2007;**15**:191–7. doi: 10.1016/s1472-6483(10)60708-0

29. Tabibnejad N, Soleimani M, Aflatoonian A. Zona pellucida birefringence and meiotic spindle visualization are not related to the time-lapse detected embryo morphokinetics in women with polycystic ovarian syndrome. *Eur J Obstet Gynecol Reprod Biol* 2018;**230**:96–102. doi: 10.1016/j.ejogrb.2018.09.029

30. de Santis L, Cino I, Rabellotti R, et al. Polar body morphology and spindle imaging as predictors of oocyte quality. *Reprod Biomed Online* 2005;**11**(1):36–42. doi: 10.1016/s1472-6483(10)61296-5

31. Ciotti PM, Notarangelo L, Morselli-Labate AM, et al. First polar body morphology before ICSI is not related to embryo quality or pregnancy rate. *Hum Reprod* 2004;**19**(10):2334–9. doi: 10.1093/humrep/deh433

32. van de Velde H, de Vos A, Joris H, Nagy ZP, van Steirteghem AC. Effect of timing of oocyte denudation and microinjection on survival, fertilization and embryo quality after intracytoplasmic sperm injection. *Hum Reprod* 1998;**13**(11):3160–4. doi: 10.1093/humrep/13.11.3160

33. Farhi J, Nahum H, Weissman A, et al. Coarse granulation in the perivitelline space and IVF-ICSI outcome. *J Assist Reprod Genet* 2002;**19**(12):545–9. doi: 10.1023/a:1021243530358

34. Rienzi L, Gajta G, Ubaldi F. Predictive value of oocyte morphology in human IVF: a systematic review of the literature *Hum Reprod Update* 2011;**17** (1):34–45. doi: 10.1093/humupd/dmq029

35. Sa R, Cunha M, Silva J, et al. Ultrastructure of tubular smooth endoplasmic reticulum aggregates in human metaphase II oocytes and clinical implications. *Fertil Steril* 2011;**96**(1):143–9.e7. doi: 10.1016/j.fertnstert.2011.04.088

36. Balakier H, Bouman D, Sojecki A, et al. Morphological and cytogenetic analysis of human giant oocytes and giant embryos. *Hum Reprod* 2002;**17** (9):2394–401. doi: 10.1093/humrep/17.9.2394

37. Verlinsky Y, Lerner S, Illkevitch N, et al. Is there any predictive value of first polar body morphology for embryo genotype or developmental potential? *Reprod Biomed Online* 2003;7:336–41. doi: 10.1016/s1472-6483(10)61874-3

38. Sanchez T, Zhang M, Needleman D, Seli E. Metabolic imaging via fluorescence lifetime imaging microscopy for egg and embryo assessment. *Fertil Steril* 2019;**111**(2):212–18. doi: 10.1016/j.fertnstert.2018.12.014

39. Patrizio P, Fragouli E, Bianchi V, Borini A, Wells D. Molecular methods for selection of the ideal oocyte. *Reprod Biomed Online* 2007;**15** (3):346–53. doi: 10.1016/s1472-6483(10)60349-5

40. Racowsky C, Needleman DJ. Cumulus cell gene expression as a potential biomarker for oocyte quality. *Fertil Steril* 2018;**109**(3):438–9. doi: 10.1016/j.fertnstert.2017.12.013

41. Kort J, Behr B. Biomechanics and developmental potential of oocytes and embryos. *Fertil Steril* 2017;**108**(5):738–41. doi: 10.1016/j.fertnstert.2017.09.016

42. Keefe D, Kumar M, Kalmbach K. Oocyte competency is the key to embryo potential. *Fertil Steril* 2015;**103**(2):317–22. doi: 10.1016/j.fertnstert.2014.12.115

43. Bukowska D, Kempisty B, Piotrowska H, et al. The invasive and new non-invasive methods of mammalian oocyte and embryo quality assessment: a review. *Vet Med (Praha)* 2012;**57**(4):169–76. doi:10.17221/5913-VETMED

44. Baart EB, Macklon NS, Fauser BJ. Ovarian stimulation and embryo quality. *Reprod Biomed Online* 2009;**18**(Suppl. 2):45–50. doi: 10.1016/s1472-6483(10)60448-8

Oocyte Preparation for Conventional In Vitro Fertilisation and Intracytoplasmic Sperm Injection

Bryan Woodward

12.1 Introduction

The aim of conventional in vitro fertilisation (cIVF) and intracytoplasmic sperm injection (ICSI) treatment cycles is to help people with fertility problems achieve their dream of having healthy live offspring. Successful treatment involves many steps in order to ensure that the oocytes are safely collected and prepared, so that fertilisation can take place in vitro. Once two pronuclei form in the oocytes, each zygote then has the opportunity to develop into a pre-implantation embryo. The most viable embryo can then be selected for transfer to the uterus for implantation hopefully to take place.

This chapter will describe the different oocyte preparation methods used by clinical embryologists to optimise the chance of successful fertilisation via cIVF and ICSI.

12.2 Initial Oocyte Preparation

The initial preparation of oocytes at the time of collection should be the same regardless of the insemination technique. Oocytes are collected from follicles as cumulus–oocyte complexes (COCs). Each COC consists of the oocyte surrounded by layers of cumulus cells. During the pre-ovulatory period, the cumulus cells should have expanded from a compact cell mass into a dispersed structure of cells. Cumulus expansion enables synthesis and deposition of a mucoid intercellular matrix and influences various developmental changes during the oocyte maturation process.

Following the appropriate superovulation regime, each patient is primed for COC collection. Following a final 'trigger' injection, the COCs are ready to be collected 36 hours later. The patient is sedated/anaesthetised and the clinical team then aspirates follicular fluid (FF) from the follicles, detected via ultrasound scanning of the patient's ovaries. The FF is dispensed into sterile test tubes, which are then placed into a heated block to maintain the FF at 37°C. The tubes in the block should be easily accessible to both the clinical team and the embryologist.

The process of identifying the COCs involves the embryologist pouring the FF into sterile Petri dishes and placing each dish onto the heated stage of a stereomicroscope to systematically search for the COCs. A COC is large enough to be seen without magnification, and is often seen as a translucent mass, several millimetres in size. Where the FF is straw-coloured, the COCs are relatively easy to detect. As the collection continues, the FF inevitably mixes with blood and becomes red in colour, with the COCs often appearing whitish in colour. Each COC should be verified using the microscope to confirm that an oocyte is present within the complex.

It is commonplace for the stereomicroscope to be fitted into a class II laminar flow hood, with the surface of the flow hood consistently heated and with an opaque aperture for the stereomicroscope light (Figure 12.1). The class II hood provides clean air throughout the COC collection to minimise the risk of contamination. The air quality for COC processing needs to be grade C against a background air quality of grade D [1], although often an air quality of grade A is achieved in class II hoods (Table 12.1).

A large heated stage enables the dishes to be pre-warmed by placing them in direct contact prior to use. Alternatively, dishes can be pre-warmed in an incubator close to the flow hood. The temperature control devices of the heated block(s), the heated stage and the incubator should ensure that the temperature of both the aspirated fluid in the tubes and the fluid in the Petri dishes is maintained at 37°C. This may require a slightly higher setting than 37°C to counter a slight heat loss during the FF transport from the follicle to the dish.

The fluid collected in the tubes is usually a mixture of FF, blood and flush medium. Clinicians may

Table 12.1. Air quality for oocyte preparation

Manipulation of oocytes and COCs should be performed in an air quality of at least grade C environment, against an environment of at least grade D air quality. Air-quality monitoring should be used as a routine measure of quality assurance, e.g. via particle counts or the use of settle plates.	
Grade	**Monitoring method**
	Air particles (number of 0.5 µm particles/ m³)[a]
A	3,500
B	3,500
C	350,000
D	3,500,000
	Settle plates (diameter 90 mm) (cfu/ 4 hours)[b]
A	<1
B	10
C	100
D	200

A) Based on ISO 14644. B) From *Rules and Guidance for Pharmaceutical Manufacturers and Distributors*. MHRA, 2002.

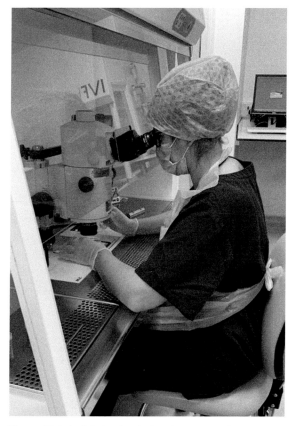

Figure 12.1 A clinical embryologist using a stereomicroscope, which has been fitted into a class II laminar flow hood. The heated surface covers the opaque aperture of the stereomicroscope to ensure all medium in dishes is maintained at 37°C. Image courtesy of the Hewitt Fertility Centre, Liverpool Women's Hospital NHS Foundation Trust, Liverpool, UK.

use a single-lumen oocyte collection needle to speed up the procedure and avoid the need for flushing [2]. However, the option of flushing may be preferred for certain patients, such as those with low follicle numbers [3].

12.3 Dish and Media Type

The dish type used for COC identification is commonly a round Petri dish. These can either be small (60 mm diameter) or large (100 mm diameter). Small dishes allow smaller volumes to be systematically checked; however, this process can use more dishes and take longer. Large dishes may allow quicker COC identification as the FF dispenses over a larger area, although there may be a quicker heat loss as a result.

Once the embryologist identifies a COC, it should be rinsed away from the surrounding FF and washed in fresh culture medium, prior to transferring to a culture dish (for a holding period prior to insemination). The culture dishes used can either be round

Petri dishes (60 mm diameter or less) or square four- or five-well dishes (Figure 12.2). Some clinics continue to use sterile tubes for culture, but these do not allow easy visualisation of the COCs compared with the use of dishes.

Some embryologists perform an initial COC wash using a culture medium buffered with either 3-(N-morpholino)propanesulfonic acid (MOPS) or 4-(2-hydroxyethyl)-1-piperazineethanesulfonic acid (HEPES), to maintain the correct pH in ambient air. Culture dishes containing MOPS- or HEPES-buffered medium should be pre-warmed to 37°C and maintained at this temperature throughout these initial steps, but never gassed. After collection, the COCs are transferred into pre-gassed medium (without MOPS or HEPES). This can reduce the time pressures at the actual time of oocyte collection, when the

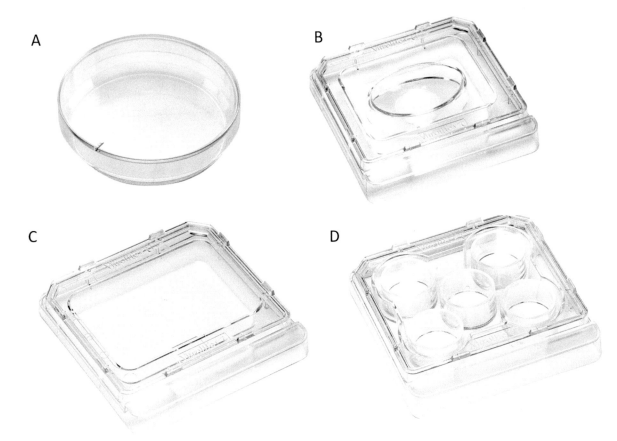

Figure 12.2 Different types of sterile dishes used for COC collection and culture. (A) Round dish. (B) Oval dish. (C) Square dish. (D) Five-well dish. Image courtesy of Vitrolife, Gothenburg, Sweden.

clinical team of nurses and clinician are aspirating the COCs.

Other clinics prefer to wash and collect the COCs directly into dishes containing a pre-gassed culture medium with a bicarbonate buffer (rather than MOPS or HEPES). Such culture dishes should be maintained in a gassed incubator, and the transfer of COCs in and out the medium should be swift, so that the COCs are always exposed to medium at the optimal pH of 7.2–7.4. If the culture medium contains phenol red, this can be a useful visual indicator of the pH level at the time of collection to reassure embryologists that the correct pH level is being maintained (Figure 12.3).

12.4 Pipette Use

Manipulation of the COC, from identification through to rinsing and transfer to the final holding dish, is performed using either a sterile glass Pasteur pipette, a pastette or a sterile pipette tip fitted to a

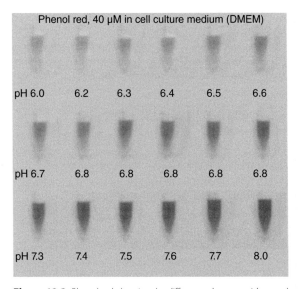

Figure 12.3 Phenol red, showing the different colours at acid, neutral and alkaline conditions. DMEM, Dulbecco's modified Eagle's medium. Image modified from Wikipedia. A black and white version of this figure will appear in some formats. For the colour version, refer to the plate section.

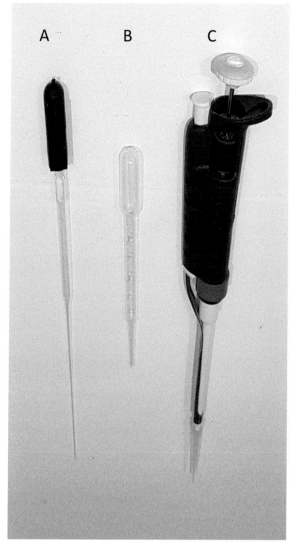

Table 12.2. Recipe for Earle's balanced salt solution

Note that this basic medium consists of only eight constituents; in contrast, the commercial IVF culture medium used today may consist of up to 80 constituents, many of which remain undisclosed by the manufacturers.

Constituent	Molecular weight	Concentration (g/L)	Molarity (mM)
NaCl	58	6.80	117.00
$NaHCO_3$	84	2.20	26.00
Glucose	180	1.00	5.56
KCl	75	0.40	5.30
$CaCl_2$	111	0.20	1.80
$NaH_2PO_4\text{-}H_2O$	120	0.14	1.17
Phenol red	398	0.01	0.03
$MgSO_4$	120	0.097	0.80

Adapted from Sigma Aldrich Datasheet E6132, www.sigmaaldrich .com/content/dam/sigma-aldrich/docs/Sigma/Datasheet/7/ e6132dat.pdf.

Figure 12.4 Different types of sterile pipettes used to transfer cumulus–oocyte complexes. (A) Glass Pasteur pipette. (B) Plastic pastette. (C) Pipette tip fitted to a 200 µl pipette. Image courtesy of X&Y Fertility, Leicester, UK.

200 µl pipette (Figure 12.4). This requires dexterity to ensure minimal carryover of fluid. Prior to COC collection, Pasteur pipettes should be checked under the microscope to ensure that the tips are smooth with no jagged edges/cracks. Nowadays, many commercial suppliers provide pipettes with polished tips ready to use. Some clinics prefer to pass the pipette tips through a flame immediately prior to use; however, this practice is considered outdated, as it forfeits any validation from the pipette supplier. A single pipette can be used for the whole process, although

some clinics prefer to use a fresh pipette for the final transfer to the holding dish.

Regardless of the choice of medium and pipette, post-collection, the COCs should be maintained in pre-gassed medium (without MOPS or HEPES) until the next step of the preparation for cIVF or ICSI.

12.5 Culture Media for COCs

The constituents of culture medium used to incubate COCs are based on salt solutions historically developed for mammalian cell culture (e.g. Earle's balanced salt solution (EBSS), Table 12.2). Over the years, modifications have taken place based on the in vivo studies of reproductive tract fluid and embryo metabolism [4]. Some commercial culture medium contains up to 80 ingredients, rather than the eight in the original EBSS, and some formulations are often not fully documented, disclosed or justified [5]. Caution should therefore be taken when selecting culture medium for oocytes and embryos, as the medium has the highest potential for causing alterations in epigenetic reprograming [5].

Some embryologists prefer to culture COCs in the same medium as used for the final sperm wash and insemination. Specifically, for cIVF, it is important to have glucose present in this culture medium – this substrate is needed for sperm motility but not by the oocyte. The medium should ideally contain a protein source that is chemically defined, such as recombinant human serum albumin, to avoid batch-to-batch variation. The protein source, which makes up 10% of the medium, acts as a surfactant to prevent the COCs from sticking to the base or sides of the culture dish.

The incubation period between COC collection and insemination is usually 2–4 hours, which is significantly less than the 5-day period between fertilisation and pre-implantation development of a blastocyst. Furthermore, the COC offers a level of protection, buffering the oocyte from direct exposure to the medium. It is a different story once the oocyte is removed from the protection of the cumulus cells, when it is more vulnerable to the medium. Adverse culture at this stage may impact on the oocyte's ability to support fertilisation and pre-implantation development, so the utmost care is required. This is why denudation for ICSI should take place as close as possible to the time of the actual ICSI process to limit exposure.

12.6 Lessons from Transport IVF

Transport IVF involves COCs being collected from patients in one clinic and then transported to another better-resourced clinic with an IVF laboratory, which is often quite a geographical distance away. COCs are collected into HEPES-buffered medium supplemented with 10% human serum albumin, in tight-capped sterile tubes, and transported in a portable incubator at 37°C to the main clinic (Figure 12.5). If we consider the practice of transport IVF, it seems that, provided the pH and temperature are kept stable, and the oocytes are maintained in healthy COCs in culture medium, oocyte viability can be adequately maintained for the time period from COC collection to insemination.

A typical transport IVF programme operates in Argentina, where the distance between clinics is about 60 km [6]. Data from 1990 to 2014 showed that the mean time elapsed between COC collection aspiration and culture in the main laboratory was just under 2 hours, with occasional delays of up to 4 hours due to vehicle breakdown or roadblocks. No deleterious effects were recorded for COCs with time delays. Furthermore, the mean pregnancy/collection rate for

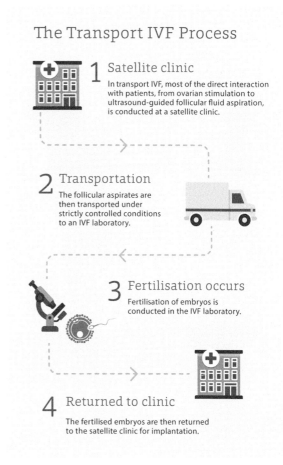

Figure 12.5 Flow diagram showing how transport IVF programmes work. Modified from Bridge Clinic, www.thebridgeclinic.com. A black and white version of this figure will appear in some formats. For the colour version, refer to the plate section.

the 25-year period was 24.7% for the transported COCs, which was not significantly different to 25.4%, the rate reported for all outcomes of Argentinian centres for the same period. Thus, for COCs, the cumulus cells offer a level of protection to the oocytes. It therefore makes sense to maintain this cell contact undisturbed until the next step of preparation.

An exception to this guidance would be if blood clots are observed to be present in the COCs. Blood clots have been associated with reduced oocyte quality (dense central granulation), fertilisation rate and blastocyst formation [7]. It could be that these COCs derive from poorer-quality follicles, which then impacts oocyte quality. Where blood clots are observed, it is advisable to carefully dissect them away to remove any potentially detrimental effects from the blood. COC processing in the subsequent preparation steps for cIVF will be significantly improved, as observation of the oocyte will be made easier.

12.7 Which Insemination Technique to Use

There are a variety of inseminating techniques available, which are all modifications of cIVF and ICSI (Table 12.3). The decision regarding the most appropriate insemination technique to use should be discussed and agreed with the patients prior to treatment. However, the final decision will depend on several factors, such as the fertilisation outcome of any previous IVF treatment, and the number of

Table 12.3. Insemination techniques historically used to promote fertilisation in human oocytes in vitro

Technique	Abbreviation	Description of technique
Conventional in vitro fertilisation	cIVF	Motile sperm are added to medium containing cumulus–oocyte complexes
Subzonal insemination	SUZI	Several motile sperm are injected into the perivitelline space
High insemination concentration	HIC	A higher than conventional concentration of motile sperm is added to medium containing oocytes
Laser-assisted in vitro fertilisation	LA-IVF	A laser is used cause several ablations through the zona pellucida; conventional IVF then takes place
Intracytoplasmic sperm injection	ICSI	A single sperm is microinjected directly into the cytoplasm of the oocyte

COCs collected and quality of the sperm sample on the day of treatment. Occasionally, after oocyte and sperm collection, it may be in the patients' best interest to change the treatment plan from cIVF to ICSI, and prepare the COCs accordingly.

12.8 Should ICSI Be Performed for All Patients?

If there is a sufficiently number of highly motile sperm of good morphology in the pre- and post-preparation stages, then the chance of fertilisation following cIVF insemination should theoretically be high. However, despite normal sperm parameters, it has been reported that 5% of cIVF attempts result in an unpredicted failure of fertilisation, with 56% of cases having no obvious oocyte anomaly other than a complete lack of ZP–sperm binding [8]. In such instances, the cause of failed fertilisation may not be ascertained without cytogenetic analysis of the unfertilised oocyte (Table 12.4).

ICSI could be perceived as the 'fix all' to avoid failed fertilisation, and there has been a trend over recent years to perform more ICSI than IVF, as demonstrated by a recent world report from the International Committee for Monitoring Assisted Reproductive Technologies [9]. This report showed

Table 12.4. Possible causes of failed fertilisation after cIVF using good-quality sperm

Observation	Possible reason	Possible gamete at fault	
		Sperm	Oocyte
No sperm attached to ZP, no PN, 1PB	Failure of sperm to penetrate cumulus	Yes	No
	Failure of sperm to bind to ZP	Yes	Yes
Sperm attached to ZP, no PN, 1PB	Failure of sperm to penetrate ooplasm	Yes	Yes
Sperm attached to ZP, no PN, 2PB	Failure of sperm chromatin to decondense in ooplasm	Yes	No

PB, polar body; PN, pronuclei; ZP, zona pellucida.

that the ICSI:IVF ratio varied from 1.4 in Asia to 60.3 in the Middle East. However, several more recent studies have shown that ICSI does not offer any benefit over cIVF across different ovarian response categories in non-male factor infertility [10, 11].

Nevertheless, some clinics prefer to reduce the risk of having a failed fertilisation and therefore promote frequent use of ICSI rather than cIVF. This is despite the additional risks associated with the ICSI procedure.

12.9 Timing of Insemination

Oocytes should be inseminated when they are thought to be at their optimal competence in terms of meiotic and cytoplasmic maturity. For COCs allocated to cIVF, this will be when the cumulus and oocyte are at their most receptive to sperm penetration and fertilisation.

Traditionally, the insemination time is based on the number of hours elapsed from the time of administration of the trigger injection (hours post-trigger). If the oocyte collection takes place at around 36 hours post-trigger, then the insemination often takes place at around 40 hours post-trigger. Some clinics perform inseminations sooner (e.g. at 38 hours post-trigger), while other clinics may choose to delay inseminations (e.g. at >40 hours post-trigger). The latter may take place if there are many immature oocytes, as indicated by the COCs having a tight unexpanded dark cumulus surrounding the oocytes (Figure 12.6). However, prediction of oocyte maturity based on COC grading is unreliable, and thus, for cIVF, all COCs should be included in the cohort for insemination [7].

Individual clinics may set their own variation in the standard timings, taking into account the number of cases and number of staff available. The embryology team may also need to adjust the timing of

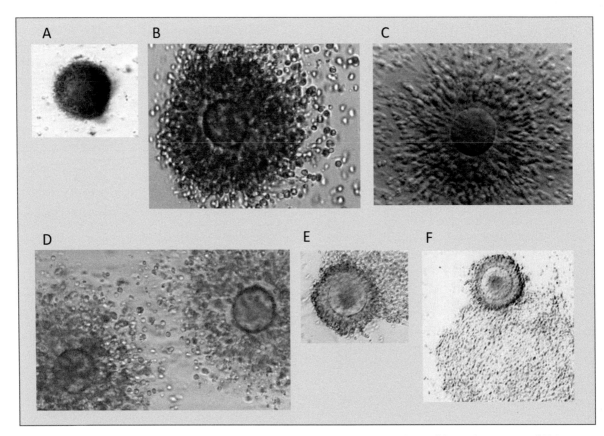

Figure 12.6 Different COCs showing immature (A, B), mature (C, D) or post-mature oocytes (E, F). While visual assessment of COCs can provide a useful indicator of maturity, it should be noted that the stage of mitosis can only truly be assessed following cumulus denudation. (A), (B), (E) and (F) courtesy of Dr Giovanna Tomasi, Centro Riproduzione Assistita s.r.l., Assisted Reproductive Center, Catania 95128, Italy; (C) and (D) courtesy of Dr Liliana Ramos, Department of Obstetrics and Gynecology, Division of Reproductive medicine, Radboud University Medical Centre, Nijmegen, The Netherlands.

insemination due to anticipated difficulty of ICSI cases. For example, to perform ICSI on a difficult case (e.g. 20 metaphase II (MII) oocytes with very poor-quality surgically retrieved sperm) will take longer than a simpler case (e.g. three MII oocytes with good-quality sperm). The start time for the former insemination may be brought forward as a result.

12.10 Confirming Patient Identity and Record Keeping

An identity check at the time of insemination ensures that the correct sperm is mixed with the correct COCs/oocytes. This involves both the embryologist and a witness checking that the identity of the COCs/oocytes and sperm belong to the same patients beyond a shadow of a doubt. The development of fail-safe mechanisms to prevent mix-ups is critical [12].

Records should be kept of the insemination time, the embryologist and the witness who confirms the identification. Furthermore, if the laboratory has more than one flow hood or ICSI workstation, the equipment should be identified and recorded so that the location of the insemination is uniquely traceable. For cIVF, the concentration of progressively motile sperm inseminated should be noted alongside the number of COCs in each insemination dish. For ICSI, any comments regarding specific oocytes should be recorded, such as dysmorphisms or difficult injections.

12.11 Oocyte Preparation for cIVF

For cIVF, COCs should be cultured in fertilisation medium in dishes where the insemination will take place. The final sperm sample should also be prepared in fertilisation medium. Prior to insemination, the sperm should be pre-equilibrated to the same conditions as the COCs: 37°C and the same gas levels. Use of the same medium for the prepared sperm sample and COCs ensures that there are no differences in medium constituents, pH and osmolality.

The number of motile sperm to be inseminated, and the volume, should be calculated to maximise the chance of fertilisation. For a prepared sperm sample, with a motility M (% progressively motile) and concentration C (million/ml), the volume to inseminate can be calculated using the equation:

Volume to inseminate (μl) $= 100/C \times \acute{M}$

This volume provides an insemination concentration of 100,000 progressively motile sperm to a volume of 1 ml of medium containing COCs. It should be noted that the insemination will be approximate, as the original medium volume will have changed with the addition of the COCs.

If the number of sperm is too high, the risk of polyspermy is increased, as well as a possible compromise of the oocyte due to the high levels of free radicals introduced with high sperm numbers. Conversely, if the number is too low, the oocytes may not fertilise. Typically, a sperm concentration of 100,000 progressively motile sperm/ml is recommended, although this can be as low as 20,000/ml or as high as 300,000/ml.

For the actual insemination process, a sterile tip should be fitted to a micropipette, set to the required insemination volume. The sperm sample should be removed from the incubator and placed in a hot block. The COC dish should be removed from the incubator and placed on a heated stage in a flow hood. The required volume of sperm should then be transferred via the pipette tip into the medium containing the COCs. The insemination should be directed away from the COCs, to allow the dispensed sperm to then swim towards the COCs. In theory, this allows the better-swimming sperm to reach the COC first.

Once all COCs have been inseminated, the medium can be observed at a magnification of $\times 400$ to check that the sperm are starting to penetrate the cumulus cells. The dish should then be returned to the incubator where it should remain until the time of the fertilisation check.

Differences to the cIVF insemination technique include: adding the sperm to a separate insemination dish and then adding the COCs; inseminating in large volumes or droplets; and reducing the time of COC and sperm co-incubation. The latter has been shown to improve outcomes for couples with a history of fragmented embryos, although more studies are needed to confirm the efficacy of this approach [13].

12.12 Oocyte Preparation for ICSI

12.12.1 Denudation of Cumulus–Corona Cells

Denudation involves disaggregating the COC by removing the cumulus–corona cells to enable visualisation of the oocyte and oolemma in detail. This is

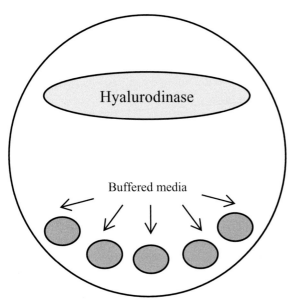

Hyalurodinase

Buffered media

Figure 12.7 Setting up a dish for oocyte denudation. The denudation dish consists of one large droplet of hyaluronidase and several smaller droplets of buffered medium (HEPES or MOPS). The COCs are initially transferred to the hyaluronidase droplets using a sterile Pasteur pipette. Once the majority of the cumulus has been removed, each oocyte with its remaining layers of cumulus cells is transferred through the wash droplet for further denudation.

performed via chemical (hyaluronidase) and mechanical (pipettes) processing.

Droplets of hyaluronidase should be prepared under oil, with wash droplets of buffered medium (e.g. HEPES or MOPS) included in the same dish (Figure 12.7). Once at 37°C, COCs should be transferred to the hyaluronidase using a sterile Pasteur pipette. They should be gently mixed with the hyaluronidase by flushing up and down the pipette. This process loosens the cumulus cells, such that the oocytes usually remain with a few layers of more tightly bound cumulus cells attached. The oocytes should then be transferred to wash droplets for further denudation.

Oocyte exposure to hyaluronidase should be kept to a minimum (30 seconds), as excessive exposure to the acid may damage oocyte ultrastructure [14]. The hyaluronidase concentration in ready-to-use media for cumulus cell removal is generally 80 IU/ml, but a diluted concentration of 30–40 IU/ml may be preferred.

Once in the wash droplets, denudation pipettes of decreasing lumen diameter (290, 190, 155 and 135 μm) should be used to remove further cumulus cells. Dedicated pipettes and pipette holders specifically designed for oocyte handling should be used. Vigorous pipetting and small pipette diameters should be avoided to prevent oocyte damage. Once fully denuded, oocyte maturation can be assessed. Incomplete oocyte denudation prior to ICSI has been suggested to possibly have benefits to oocyte quality [15]. However, it is essential that there is sufficient cytoplasm that is clearly visible to allow accurate assessment of the oocyte maturity.

12.12.2 Assessing Oocytes Prior to ICSI

Post-denudation, it is useful to document the maturity and any obvious defects of the oocytes. For example, for maturity, the number of oocytes at II should be recorded, along with the number of oocytes at other stages (metaphase I (MI), germinal vesicle). General dysmorphisms should also be noted, such as the number of oocytes with abnormal shape or possessing a fragmented or giant polar body. Large oocytes and immature germinal vesicle-stage oocytes can be discarded at this stage. MII oocytes should be washed in pre-equilibrated culture medium and incubated prior to ICSI. MI oocytes should also be kept, in case they mature to MII by the time of ICSI [16]. MI oocytes may also be left overnight to allow them to mature, but this practice is less common.

Oocyte quality can also be assessed prior to ICSI by using computerised polarisation microscopy, which allows digital imaging of birefringent structures such as the zona pellucida and meiotic spindle [17]. The level of birefringence may then be used to help grade oocyte quality and to predict the potential of any embryos that subsequently develop. However, others have questioned the usefulness of this technology [18].

12.13 Summary

This chapter has outlined the techniques involved for preparing oocytes in vitro for either cIVF or ICSI. Practical advice on methods, including tips for optimising outcomes and troubleshooting have been provided. Clinical embryologists who wish to read more about COC and oocyte quality are recommended to read atlases on embryology, such as the web version of the *Atlas of Embryology* produced by the European Society of Human Reproduction and Embryology accessible from PC, tablets and smartphones and having open access at the time of writing (https:// atlas.eshre.eu/).

References

1. Commission of the European Parliament. *Directive 2004/23/EC of the European Parliament and of the Council of 31 March 2004 on Setting Standards of Quality and Safety for the Donation, Procurement, Testing, Processing, Preservation, Storage and Distribution of Human Tissues and Cells.* Brussels: European Union, 2004. https://eur-lex .europa.eu/LexUriServ/ LexUriServ.do?uri=OJ: L:2004:102:0048:0058:en:PDF

2. Georgiou EX, Melo P, Brown J, Granne IE Follicular flushing during oocyte retrieval in assisted reproductive techniques. *Cochrane Database Syst Rev* 2018;**4**:CD004634. doi: 10.1002/ 14651858.CD004634.pub3

3. ESHRE Working Group on Ultrasound in ART. Recommendations for good practice in Ultrasound: oocyte pick-up. *Hum Reprod Open* 2019;**2019**(4):hoz025. doi: 10.1093/hropen/hoz025

4. Leese HJ. History of oocyte and embryo metabolism. *Reprod Fertil Dev* 2015;**27**(4):567–71. doi: 10.1071/RD14278

5. Sunde A, Brison D, Dumoulin J, et al. Time to take human embryo culture seriously. *Hum Reprod* 2016;**31**(10):2174–82. doi: 10.1093/humrep/dew157

6. Raffo FGE, Blaquier J. Transport IVF-ICSI: Results of a 25-year experience. *JBRA Assist Reprod* 2018;**22**(2):123–7. doi: 10.5935/ 1518-0557.20180026

7. Ebner T, Moser M, Shebl O, et al. Blood clots in the cumulus–oocyte complex predict poor oocyte quality and post-fertilization development. *Reprod Biomed Online* 2008;**16**(6):801–7. doi: 10.1016/s1472-6483(10)60145-9.

8. Frapsauce C, Pionneau C, Bouley J, et al. [Unexpected in vitro fertilisation failure in patients with normal sperm: a proteomic analysis.] *Gynecol Obstet Fertil* 2009;**37**(10):796–802. doi: 10.1016/j.gyobfe.2009.07.014

9. Dyer S, Chambers GM, de Mouzon J, et al. International Committee for Monitoring Assisted Reproductive Technologies world report: Assisted Reproductive Technology 2008, 2009 and 2010. *Hum Reprod* 2016;**31** (7):1588–609. doi: 10.1093/ humrep/dew082

10. Drakopoulos P, Garcia-Velasco J, Bosch E, et al. Correction to: ICSI does not offer any benefit over conventional IVF across different ovarian response categories in non-male factor infertility: a European multicenter analysis. *J Assist Reprod Genet* 2019;**36** (10):2077–8. doi: 10.1007/s10815-019-01586-8

11. Gennarelli G, Carosso A, Canosa S, et al. ICSI versus conventional IVF in women aged 40 years or more and unexplained infertility: a retrospective evaluation of 685 cycles with propensity score model. *J Clin Med* 2019;**8** (10):1694. doi: 10.3390/ jcm8101694

12. Rienzi L, Bariani F, Dalla Zorza M, et al. Comprehensive protocol of traceability during IVF: the result of a multicentre failure mode and effect analysis. *Hum Reprod* 2017;**32**(8):1612–20. doi: 10.1093/humrep/dex144

13. Le Bras A, Hesters L, Gallot V, et al. Shortening gametes co-incubation time improves live birth rate for couples with a history of fragmented embryos. *Syst Biol Reprod Med* 2017;**63** (5):331–7. doi: 10.1080/ 19396368.2017.1336581

14. de Vos A, van Landuyt L, van Ranst H, et al. Randomized sibling–oocyte study using recombinant human hyaluronidase versus bovine-derived Sigma hyaluronidase in ICSI patients. *Hum Reprod* 2008;**23**(8):1815–19. doi: 10.1093/ humrep/den212

15. Ebner T, Moser M, Sommergruber M, Shebl O, Tews G Incomplete denudation of oocytes prior to ICSI enhances embryo quality and blastocyst development. *Hum Reprod* 2006;**21**(11):2972–7. doi: 10.1093/ humrep/del272

16. Montag M, Schimming T, van der Ven H. Spindle imaging in human oocytes: the impact of the meiotic cell cycle. *Reprod Biomed Online* 2006;**12**(4):442–6. doi: 10.1016/s1472-6483(10) 61996-7.

17. Dib LA, Araújo MC, Giorgenon RC, et al. Noninvasive imaging of the meiotic spindle of in vivo matured oocytes from infertile women with endometriosis. *Reprod Sci* 2013;**20** (4):456–62. doi: 10.1177/ 1933719112459217

18. Swiatecka J, Bielawski T, Anchim T, et al. Oocyte zona pellucida and meiotic spindle birefringence as a biomarker of pregnancy rate outcome in IVF-ICSI treatment. *Ginekol Pol* 2014;**85**(4):264–71. doi: 10.17772/gp/1722

Chapter 13

Oocyte Retrieval: The Patient's Perspective

Kate Brian

13.1 Introduction

From the patient's perspective, egg collection is the focal point of in vitro fertilisation (IVF) or intracytoplasmic sperm injection, often following many years of fertility problems, tests and other treatments. This is the moment at which there is an indication of the chances of success, depending on the number of eggs harvested, and many patients experience a combination of excitement and anxiety as egg collection approaches. It can be a nerve-wracking time, and clinicians can help to improve the patient's experience of this stage of fertility treatment by appreciating the emotions involved, recognising the impact they can have and acting with empathy towards their patients.

The emotional significance of egg collection for a fertility patient cannot be underestimated as the culmination of the weeks of preparation approaches. This patient explained, 'When I was having my eggs collected I felt really special. I was often aware of the other women in the clinic, and I was thinking I'd got to the grown up bit' [1]. Egg collection is such a key part of treatment for a patient that there is often an expectation that the clinical team should show the kind of respect for the occasion their patient may feel it deserves. The fact that this does not always happen is one of a number of themes that emerge from discussions with patients about their experiences of egg collection. There are some areas that merit consideration by those working in fertility clinics where there may be room to improve practice.

13.2 Information

It is clear that, despite the plethora of information available about egg collection for patients, they may still feel uncertain about what to expect on the day itself. Many patients will carry out their own

---

Unattributed quotes are from interviews with the author.

independent research online alongside the written and verbal information they have been given about egg collection by their clinic, and are likely to have read about other people's experiences. This can be useful but may sometimes serve to increase anxiety rather than reduce it, as those posting online may be doing so because something unusual or untoward has happened during or after their own egg collection. This can lead to worries about complications such as ovarian hyperstimulation syndrome (OHSS), pain or the possibility of a less-than-positive outcome.

When I went to the clinic for egg collection during my first IVF cycle, I had read every last word of the information I had been given by my clinic, and a number of books on the subject. Despite this, I still had a vision of egg collection as 'some kind of glorified smear test' and it wasn't until I arrived at hospital on the day that I realised it was 'more of a minor operation than a major smear test' [2]. Even now, when patients have much more information available to them, some are still left confused, as this patient explains: 'I had been quite anxious about the egg retrieval. I thought it would be very painful. I hadn't actually realised until about a week before that they took the eggs out through the vaginal wall' [3].

Patients may arrive at their clinics for egg collection with last-minute anxieties or questions that have been unanswered, and often feel unsure who they should address them to. If a clinic has made an effort to ensure that they have given their patients as much information about egg collection as they can, and has explained who their patients should turn to with any queries in advance or on the day, this will help them to approach egg collection feeling less anxious and worried.

13.3 Waiting for Egg Collection

One common concern for patients is the waiting that often happens at the clinic on the morning of egg collection. They are very aware that timing is vitally important when it comes to this part of their fertility treatment, and if they are asked to come into the clinic fairly early in the morning, they assume this is because it is necessary for their treatment rather than necessary to make things easier for the clinic staff. If they are then left sitting about with no clear explanation as to why, or any reassurance that this is normal rather than an indication of a problem on the day, it can raise levels of anxiety, as this patient explained to me: 'The waiting before we had egg collection was one of the most difficult parts of the entire day. We were left in this cubicle, just the two of us left sitting there for what seemed like hours. It made me feel more and more anxious as I was really worried they had just forgotten all about us and that it was going to be too late to collect my eggs.'

Ruth Wilde, fertility counsellor and former chair of the British Infertility Counselling Association, feels that fertility clinics could do more to support their patients at this stage. 'Patients often feel that they are not made a priority in the clinic when they go in for egg collection, and all the hanging around they experience does come up in complaints. It's part of the clinic organisation that everyone having egg collection needs to be in early, never mind how long the patient has to wait. This is the most important day of their treatment, but there is an issue with this about whose needs are being met.'

Many clinics provide excellent information about egg collection, but much of it focuses on the clinical aspects of treatment. What patients would often welcome alongside this is more practical information about what they can expect to happen on the day. If they are likely to be left waiting for some time, it is important to make it clear that this may occur. If they will have to share the waiting or recovery room with other patients, then explain this in advance. Patients are much less likely to be upset by these things if they are forewarned, and this can help them to feel that they are being treated as individuals and that the clinic is thinking about how the experience may feel from their point of view.

13.4 Pain during Egg Collection

Concerns about pain during egg collection are common, and patients are not always clear about what kind of pain relief they will be getting. Clinic information may tell them they will have a 'light general anaesthetic' or 'heavy sedation', and although it may be clear to an anaesthetist what this means, many patients are not sure what the difference is between the two or what they might expect to experience with either. Talking to other patients or reading their experiences online can serve to raise concerns, as the level of pain patients experience varies hugely from those who report being totally knocked out by sedation to others who have experienced severe pain. It is helpful if clinics are able to give clear information about the type of anaesthesia they offer and the effect it may have.

This patient's experience of anxiety about pain before egg collection is common: 'I was very worried that I'd be wide awake and know all about it, and I was anxious because there were all these follicles, but you don't know if there are any eggs in them. Actually I didn't remember a thing about it. I only remember coming round in the recovery room and asking how many eggs I had' [2]. Another said to me, 'In my mind, I'd built egg collection up into some really frightening thing. I was so scared on the day that I could feel myself trembling, but it was one of the easiest parts of IVF. It was uncomfortable when they were prodding about, and there was a bit of bleeding, but it was nothing like as bad as I expected.'

For some patients, however, the experience is less pleasant. One patient told me, 'The egg collection was painful. I can remember that very vividly. I was quite awake and I could feel things happening. It was horrible.' Another reported having to ask for additional drugs during the process: 'I was awake right through the egg collection. They were giving the sedation through a drip in my arm. I had to ask for more and they didn't seem to think I should need it. The whole thing took a really long time because there were so many follicles.'

13.5 Handing over Control

One emotional challenge for patients at this stage of treatment is the idea of handing over of control of their eggs and sperm to the clinic's embryologists. They entrust the team with their precious gametes, which they leave in the laboratory and go home with no control at all over what happens next. If at this stage they start to have doubts about the staff or the clinic, it can have a devastating impact, but they may not always have the confidence to ask the questions they want answered.

Playwright Gareth Farr touches on the loss of control patients experience after egg collection in his play about IVF, *The Quiet House* [4]. The female lead character, Jess, is explaining what will happen to her partner, Dylan. 'We hand everything over to them. We pray to the goddess of procreation that some of them are mature and able to fertilise and then they phone us one day at a time to tell us how many have survived. We pray some more and if there's some left at day five then we put one back where it belongs.' Gareth Farr deftly illustrates the powerlessness of the patient; there is nothing that Dylan and Jess can do but pray as they wait to find out what has happened.

With current witnessing technology, the chances of a mix-up in the clinic may be highly unlikely, but the fact that there have been high-profile cases where the wrong gametes have been used, or the wrong embryos have been transferred, leads to an inevitable underlying anxiety for some patients. In her book *The Pursuit of Motherhood*, author Jessica Hepburn explains how she insisted on witnessing the sperm preparation for her intrauterine insemination treatment herself due to her fear of her partner's sperm being mixed up with someone else's. The clinic staff allowed her to watch the preparation process, but she was so distressed when the sperm arrived in a different tube for the insemination that she refused to go ahead with the treatment cycle [5]. Although it may be unusual for a patient to request this, many will be wishing they could keep an eye on what happens to their gametes when they are in the laboratory. Patient information that explains how carefully eggs, sperm and embryos are cared for at the clinic and that attempts to demystify the processes that take place in the laboratory is beneficial to patients.

13.6 The Pressure on the Male Partner

The attention at this stage of treatment is usually focused on the woman having her eggs collected, but unless donor or frozen sperm is being used, the male partner is under considerable pressure to produce his sample to ensure the cycle can proceed smoothly. Men may not easily admit to any worries about this, and one nurse explained that men find it hard to talk about their concerns throughout the treatment process. 'Men struggle so much during treatment, and not many men can say "I am finding this hard and I don't like it"' [2].

Fertility counsellor Ruth Wilde told me the anxiety men feel on egg collection day is often completely overlooked: 'The lack of attention to partners is a significant concern. They don't know what their role is and often aren't told where they are meant to be or where they are allowed to go in the clinic. They have to give their sperm sample on the day, and the pressure and anxiety around that is huge. They not only have their own anxiety about this but also feel the need to support their partner on the day, and that is often difficult for them.'

One female patient told me that her partner didn't admit how anxious he was about the quality of his sample until the eggs had fertilised: 'When the embryologist called and told us we had six embryos, my husband burst into tears. I hadn't realised how stressed and worried he'd been about whether it was going to work and whether it was going to be OK. He was absolutely beside himself. He'd been so fraught and worried that his sperm wasn't going to be good enough and that we wouldn't get any embryos.' Recognition that the male partner may also be finding this tough and treating him with empathy will be helpful.

13.7 Care and Dignity

Many women report that they find the entire process of egg collection undignified, and this may be exacerbated when they sense that there is a lack of sensitivity to their feelings. If women are left waiting for long periods dressed in hospital gowns feeling unsure of what happens next, if clinicians do not seem to be treating them with respect and empathy, or if they don't feel they are being treated as individuals, this can all add to the sense of indignity, as this patient explained to me: 'They were just chatting away to one another while I was lying there, and it didn't seem as if they were thinking about me or how I might be feeling at all.'

For patients, egg collection is an important occasion, a key part of their treatment, and when they are not treated with dignity and respect, it can make them start to feel worried about wider aspects of a clinic's care. It does not need any additional time or emotional investment to treat patients with dignity and respect during treatment. This is really just a matter of treating them as you would like to be treated yourself. Being kind and showing that you are thinking of them as individuals will affect the way they feel about the care they receive at the clinic.

13.8 Calling Out the Number of Eggs

Some patients are aware of the team calling out when they find an egg in the fluid from the follicles. This isn't always easy, as one patient explained to me: 'For me, the most difficult bit was hearing them count the eggs as they collected them. I hadn't responded well to the drugs, so I was just desperately hoping we had enough eggs and I hadn't expected to hear them shouting it out like that.'

Another found this part of treatment a challenge as it made her very aware of her infertility, and of the sadness of her situation. 'We went into a room where there was a bed with stirrupy contraptions which looked sadly like everything you've been brought up to think of as a birth bed... Then you get, "Yes, it's an egg, it's an egg." It's a bit like your version of "It's a boy" or "It's a girl", but it's just a load of eggs. I remember crying a bit because it suddenly struck me that there I was with [my husband] mopping my brow, and the nurse saying "It's OK, it won't be long." It was exactly the scene you picture with birth, though I was giving birth to five microscopic eggs' [1].

13.9 Delivering Results

From a clinical point of view, it is an unfortunate but not uncommon experience for a patient to end up with fewer eggs than expected after egg collection, or even to discover that there are no eggs at all. For the patient, this is an absolutely devastating blow. There has been a long build-up to this point in treatment and patients have already endured considerable emotional distress. If there are no eggs, or fewer than the patient had hoped for, it is important to bear in mind the need to deal with delivering bad news sensitively. This patient told me about her response: 'I remember crying when they said there were only three eggs. There had been so many follicles but hardly any of them contained eggs. When I came round I kept asking, "How may eggs? How many eggs?" and I burst into tears when they told me. I was so emotional about everything.'

Fertility counsellor Ruth Wilde says this is an area where clinics could improve on their practice. 'When it comes to egg collection, people are often recovering in the same room as others who have also just had their eggs collected. There is very little privacy and every conversation with their partner is a whisper. I was horrified that a patient who was told she had no eggs was put opposite a woman who had 12. She

was told this by the consultant in such a matter of fact way that she didn't feel she could make a fuss. With any other bad news, there is some kind of ceremony, but this is often said with scant regard for how catastrophic it can feel to a patient – and people are not prepared. The way news is given either gives people permission to be upset or it doesn't, and bad news is often delivered in a way that doesn't in fertility clinics.'

It should be expected that any patient receiving bad news after egg collection will be extremely upset and will need care and support. Clinics should think about how they deal with this eventuality, and recognise the impact it may have on the patient.

13.10 Post-retrieval

It is always helpful if clinicians give patients some idea of what to expect after egg collection. Of course, there are patients who experience no side effects at all, but others may experience discomfort, spotting, cramping or soreness. If they are aware that they may experience some side effects, this can really help, as this patient explained to me: 'They did tell us I might feel really uncomfortable afterwards and explained about potential side effects. As it was, I felt so well that I got up the next day and was out and about.' However, for those who are not prepared, it can be more worrying: 'I had really bad bloating and terrible constipation, and had to take pain killers to get through the day and to allow me to go to sleep at night. It lasted for quite a few days which I hadn't expected at all.'

Most patients are aware of OHSS and know it can be a potentially dangerous side effect of ovarian stimulation, but the severity of the symptoms of what is classified as mild OHSS can come as a surprise, as this patient explained to me: 'It was a few days after embryo transfer that my stomach started swelling up. I started to really panic. I went into hospital and they said it was mild OHSS, but it was really uncomfortable and I couldn't sleep at all.'

Women who experience more severe OHSS find it to be an unpleasant and often frightening experience. 'I was pretty aware that something was wrong. I was feeling really sick and hormonal with mood swings and headaches, and every time they scanned me, they could see there were a lot of eggs. You just swell up because you are retaining so much fluid and I ended up in hospital. There was this one evening when I'd been feeling pretty awful and I was suddenly swelling.

I'm usually a size eight and my waist was 34 inches. I'd gained five pounds in an hour. I had to stay in overnight and it did stabilise. I felt completely rotten about the whole thing as I kept thinking I am not just ill, but I am actually doing this to myself.'

For some patients, there can be very real dangers to their health. 'I started being sick, and I felt so swollen I could hardly stand. I was admitted to hospital and my weight was going up about half a stone every day. My legs filled up with fluid too and I was mortified. I was in hospital for 2 weeks. They were monitoring me every day, checking my urine, and they had to drain off the fluid. I think my husband was more frightened because when you're the patient, you just accept it. I don't think I realised how near I was to it becoming a disastrous situation. What finished it off was that out of the 26 eggs, only one fertilised.'

It is important that patients know who they can contact if they have any worrying side effects directly after egg collection, and ideally they should have a name as well as a contact number. They should be aware of how they might feel after egg collection, and what should lead them to call the clinic or seek medical help right away. They should be made to feel that it would be fine to call if they have concerns, and that any worries will be treated with understanding and a supportive attitude.

13.11 Waiting and Anxiety

Patients are usually told that the clinic will phone them to let them know whether their eggs have fertilised. Waiting for this call is one of the most challenging phases of the cycle, and if clinics are able to be clear about when they will be calling, this can help, as any unexpected delay adds to the anxiety. These calls mark the moment patients will discover whether they have got through to the final stage of treatment, and most spend the day entirely focused on the phone. 'I was waiting for the embryologist to call and that was really tough. I couldn't think about anything else and it was such a worrying time. I was really anxious and I felt uncomfortable from the egg collection so all I could do was sit in bed. Just sitting around not doing anything means you think about it even more, and I was just so worried waiting for that call.'

Clinics are aware of the importance of this moment for their patients, and calls can be challenging to make if the outcome is less positive than

anticipated. It is important to remember the impact this will have on a patient who has been through a huge amount both emotionally and physically, and who may also be under immense financial pressure if the cycle is self-funded. A disappointing outcome signals the loss of hope for this cycle but may also mark the loss of hope of ever having a child of their own if this is the end of their treatment.

Although patients may know it is theoretically possible that their eggs will not fertilise, most do not expect that this will happen to them. If there have been a number of eggs and good-quality sperm, not having any embryos can come as a real shock, as this patient explained to me: 'The sperm on the day was fantastic and there was nothing wrong with the eggs. We don't know why they didn't fertilise. We left the clinic with such positive feedback. Everything was looking great, the sperm were really good, the eggs were really good, we were young and I'd been pregnant before. When they rang the next day to say nothing had fertilised, that was one of my very lowest points and the next 6 months were just awful. There was nothing to indicate it might happen. They said it was just one of those things.'

13.12 Grading of Embryos

Patients are often given a grade for their embryos once they have been collected, but they do not always know what the grading means, particularly as not all clinics do this the same way. It is not an issue if they are told their embryos are top quality, but confusion arises more often around lower gradings and what this means in practice. There are sometimes concerns that transferring an embryo that is not top grade may lead to problems for any future child, as this patient explained: 'We were told that they weren't really the best embryos, but they were pregnancy grade. I thought, what does that mean? Does that mean the baby will come out with one arm missing? There's so much that's not explained, and then when you go looking, you're often told they don't really know' [2].

13.13 To Blastocyst or Not

With the growing trend towards single blastocyst transfer, many patients will be hoping to go for a later embryo transfer. Sometimes, there are not sufficient good-quality embryos to go to the blastocyst stage, or an embryologist may give clear guidance that there are a number of good-quality embryos and the patient can feel confident about waiting, but where there is any ambiguity, it can be difficult for patients to decide what to do. Of course, some are very determined about what they want, regardless of any advice. One woman told me: 'They said they were worried there might not be any left if we went to day 5, but I said I wanted to take the chance. They said the embryos didn't meet their eligibility criteria as they weren't good quality, but I said it was my decision.'

Although the final decision should be made by the patient, it needs to be well informed. It is essential that clinics provide all the help and guidance they can for patients about why they are recommending a particular route.

13.14 Fertility Preservation

Not all women undergoing egg collection will be expecting to have an embryo transfer in the same cycle. Some may be going through the process for fertility preservation, either because they have a medical condition or they are having treatment that may affect their fertility. Others may be freezing eggs because they want to increase their chances of having a child later in life. In these cases, the number of eggs is vital, as many women may know from the outset that they will not be able to have another cycle, for either medical or financial reasons. For some, there may be bigger questions about their own health if they are having egg collection before cancer treatment, and it is important that healthcare professionals are mindful of the circumstances of these patients when caring for them after egg collection.

13.15 Egg Donors

The other category of women who often get overlooked are those who are donating their eggs, either as altruistic donors or as egg sharers. For egg sharers,

the number of eggs will be crucial, but those who are donating are also hoping to provide the recipient with the best chance of pregnancy possible, and can be very upset if they don't get the number of eggs they were hoping for.

There is often very little in the way of after-care for egg donors, and fertility counsellor Ruth Wilde told me that this is another area where care could be improved: 'The egg donors don't come back to clinic so it is more important they get followed up. It is not routine to call them, and they are usually told just to get in touch if they have a concern, but the clinic should be actively checking that they are OK and thanking them, especially when they may be in pain, and acknowledging just how wonderful what they've done is.'

13.16 Summary

An understanding of the importance that egg collection has for patients and a recognition of this from clinics in the information they provide and the way they offer care at this time can make all the difference to the experience. Giving clear information about practicalities as well as the clinical aspects of treatment will mean your patients know what to expect, and this can help with the feelings of loss of control. It will also help ensure that they are not reliant on what may be less than accurate information that they have found themselves online. The Human Fertilisation and Embryology Authority now asks all clinics to implement a patient support policy to ensure that the emotional needs of those going through fertility treatment are addressed. Of course, clinics can be busy and staff are often rushed, but if you can still manage to convey an empathetic approach and to treat your patients as individuals, this will help your patients have confidence in you and your clinic, and to feel that they are being well cared for.

References

1. Brian K. *In Pursuit of Parenthood*. London: Bloomsbury, 1998.

2. Brian K. *The Complete Guide to IVF*. London: Piatkus, 2009.

3. Brian K. *The Complete Guide to Female Fertility*. London: Piatkus, 2007.

4. Farr G. *The Quiet House*. London: Nick Hern Books, 2016.

5. Hepburn J. *The Pursuit of Motherhood*. Market Harborough: Matador, 2014.

Index

Printed in the United States
by Baker & Taylor Publisher Services